INTRODUCTION

Polymyalgia rheumatica (PMR) is a challenging inflammatory disorder predominantly affecting individuals over 50, characterized by pain, stiffness, and inflammation in specific areas of the body, notably the shoulders, neck, hips, and thighs. The precise cause of PMR remains elusive, contributing to the complexity of diagnosis and treatment. While medical interventions play a central role in managing PMR, lifestyle factors, particularly diet, are increasingly recognized as a potential influencer of symptoms and overall well-being.

This exploration delves into the intricacies of PMR, examining its clinical manifestations, the impact on daily life, and the evolving understanding of how dietary choices may contribute to its management. As we unravel the complexities of this condition, we embark on a journey to understand the symbiotic relationship between inflammatory processes, nutritional elements, and the body's response to both.

The intersection of PMR and diet is a dynamic field, with emerging research shedding light on the potential benefits of specific foods in mitigating inflammation and improving symptoms. From anti-inflammatory properties found in certain fruits and vegetables to the potential impact of dietary habits on the overall inflammatory burden, this guide seeks to empower individuals with PMR with the knowledge to make informed choices about their diet.

Recognizing that each individual's experience with PMR is unique, incorporating dietary considerations into a holistic management approach warrants careful and individualized attention. This guide aims to navigate the intricate landscape of PMR and diet, fostering an understanding that goes beyond mere sustenance to explore how nutritional choices can complement conventional treatments, contributing to a more personalized approach to wellness.

In the following pages, we delve into the scientific underpinnings of PMR, the potential links between inflammation and dietary patterns, and practical insights into making nutritional choices that align with individual health goals. Through this exploration, we aim to provide individuals with PMR the tools to participate in their well-being actively. We offer a nuanced understanding of how diet can be a valuable ally in managing this challenging condition.

CHAPTER ONE

Defining Polymyalgia Rheumatica (PMR)

Polymyalgia rheumatica (PMR) stands as a distinctive and challenging inflammatory syndrome primarily affecting individuals over the age of 50, with a predilection for those in their 70s and 80s. Characterized by a symmetrical pattern of pain and stiffness, PMR predominantly targets the shoulders, neck, hips, and thighs, significantly impacting daily activities and diminishing overall quality of life.

ETIOLOGY AND RISK FACTORS

Polymyalgia rheumatica (PMR) remains an enigmatic inflammatory disorder, and its precise etiology continues to elude the medical community. This condition is likely multifactorial and influenced by a combination of genetic, environmental, and immunologic factors. Although the exact triggers remain uncertain, several potential causes and risk factors have been identified, shedding light on the intricate landscape of PMR.

1. Age and Gender:

    PMR predominantly affects individuals over the age of 50, with the highest incidence seen in those in their 70s and 80s. This age-related susceptibility suggests a potential link between aging processes and the development of PMR.

    Women are more commonly affected than men, with a female-to-male ratio of approximately 2:1. The reasons for this gender disparity remain under investigation.

2. Genetic Predisposition:

    There is evidence to suggest a genetic component in the development of PMR, as individuals with a family history of autoimmune diseases or inflammatory conditions may be at an increased risk.

Specific genetic markers and variations in immune-related genes have been explored for potential associations with PMR susceptibility.

3. Inflammatory and Immunologic Factors:

PMR is characterized by systemic inflammation, and an overactive immune response is believed to contribute to its pathogenesis. The exact triggers initiating this immune response have yet to be fully understood.

Infections, particularly viral infections, have been hypothesized as potential triggers for PMR, although conclusive evidence linking specific infections to the development of the condition is lacking.

4. Environmental Factors:

Geographic variations in PMR incidence rates have been observed, suggesting a potential role for environmental factors. However, no specific environmental triggers have been definitively identified.

Some studies have explored the impact of seasonal changes and climate on PMR, but the results are inconclusive.

5. Giant Cell Arteritis (GCA) Connection:

PMR and Giant Cell Arteritis (GCA) often coexist, and individuals diagnosed with one condition are at an increased risk of developing the other. This association highlights shared pathogenic mechanisms between the two disorders.

6. Hormonal Influences:

Hormonal factors, such as changes in hormonal levels during aging or menopause, have been proposed as potential contributors to PMR. The higher prevalence of PMR in women and the occurrence around the age of menopause suggest a hormonal influence.

SYMPTOMS OF POLYMYALGIA RHEUMATICA (PMR)

Here are the symptoms associated with PMR:

1. Pain and Stiffness:

> Predominantly in Shoulders and Hips: One of the cardinal symptoms of PMR is bilateral pain and stiffness, particularly in the shoulders and hips. This discomfort is often more pronounced in the morning or after periods of inactivity, making daily activities challenging.

2. Symmetrical Involvement:

> Bilateral Pattern: PMR exhibits a symmetrical distribution of symptoms, meaning that both sides of the body are affected equally. This symmetrical involvement is a critical feature that helps distinguish PMR from other conditions.

3. Morning Stiffness:

> Profound Upon Waking: Stiffness tends to be most severe in the morning, leading to difficulty initiating movements. As the day progresses and individuals engage in more activity, stiffness

gradually diminishes.

4. Generalized Aches:

Neck and Torso: Beyond the shoulders and hips, PMR-induced pain and stiffness may extend to the neck and torso, impacting the ability to perform routine tasks and compromising overall mobility.

5. Fatigue and Malaise:

Generalized Weakness: Individuals with PMR often experience pervasive fatigue and a sense of malaise, contributing to an overall feeling of weakness and decreased energy levels.

6. Weight Loss:

Unintentional: Unexplained weight loss is a potential symptom of PMR. This could be a result of the systemic impact of inflammation and the associated metabolic changes.

7. Fever and Night Sweats:

Occasional Fever: Some individuals with PMR may experience low-grade fevers, especially during periods of active inflammation. Night sweats may also occur, contributing to sleep disturbances.

8. Limited Range of Motion:

Impaired Mobility: The pain and stiffness associated with PMR can lead to a limited range of motion in affected joints, significantly impacting daily activities such as dressing, reaching, and lifting.

9. Depression and Anxiety:

Psychological Impact: The chronic nature of PMR, coupled with the physical limitations it imposes, can contribute to emotional distress. Depression and anxiety may be secondary symptoms in some individuals.

10. Temporal Artery Symptoms (in association with Giant Cell Arteritis):

Headaches and Scalp Tenderness: Individuals with PMR may also experience symptoms related to Giant Cell Arteritis, such as headaches and tenderness over the temporal arteries.

DIAGNOSIS OF POLYMYALGIA RHEUMATICA (PMR)

Polymyalgia rheumatica (PMR) presents a diagnostic challenge due to its complex and overlapping symptoms with other inflammatory conditions. The diagnostic process requires a meticulous evaluation involving a combination of clinical assessment, laboratory tests, and imaging studies. This overview illuminates the intricacies of diagnosing PMR, aiming to empower both healthcare professionals and individuals on the journey toward an accurate and timely diagnosis.

1. Clinical Evaluation:

> Detailed Medical History: The diagnostic journey typically commences with a thorough medical history, wherein healthcare professionals explore the onset, duration, and progression of symptoms. Particular attention is paid to the pattern of pain and stiffness, emphasizing the symmetrical involvement of shoulders, hips, and other joints.

> Physical Examination: A comprehensive physical examination is paramount, focusing on joint assessments, range of motion, and the presence

of characteristic symptoms such as shoulder and hip pain. Particular attention may be given to identifying signs associated with Giant Cell Arteritis, a condition that often coexists with PMR.

2. Laboratory Tests:

Elevated Inflammatory Markers: Blood tests play a crucial role in the diagnosis of PMR. Elevations in inflammatory markers, including erythrocyte sedimentation rate (ESR) and C-reactive protein (CRP), are frequently observed in individuals with PMR. These markers reflect the extent of inflammation in the body.

Complete Blood Count (CBC): An analysis of the complete blood count may reveal anemia, which is common in individuals with PMR.

3. Imaging Studies:

Ultrasound and MRI: Imaging studies, such as ultrasound and magnetic resonance imaging (MRI), may be employed to assess the degree of inflammation in affected joints and soft tissues. These studies can provide valuable insights into the extent of involvement and help rule out other conditions mimicking PMR.

Temporal Artery Biopsy: A temporal artery biopsy may be recommended if Giant Cell Arteritis is suspected. This procedure involves removing and examining a small segment of the temporal artery to detect inflammation.

4. Response to Treatment:

Diagnostic Criterion: A hallmark of PMR diagnosis is

the rapid and significant improvement in symptoms following the initiation of corticosteroid treatment. A positive response to low-dose corticosteroids supports the diagnosis of PMR.

5. Exclusion of Other Conditions:

Differential Diagnosis: Given the overlap of symptoms with other inflammatory and rheumatic conditions, healthcare professionals must systematically rule out alternative diagnoses. Conditions such as rheumatoid arthritis, osteoarthritis, and fibromyalgia may present with similar symptoms, necessitating a thorough evaluation to differentiate PMR.

6. Collaborative Approach:

Multidisciplinary Team: Diagnosing PMR often requires a collaborative approach involving rheumatologists, primary care physicians, and, if applicable, specialists in vascular medicine for Giant Cell Arteritis evaluation. Communication and information sharing among healthcare providers are pivotal for a comprehensive diagnostic assessment.

TREATMENT OPTIONS

Here are the various aspects of PMR treatment:

1. Corticosteroids:

> Initial Treatment: Corticosteroids, particularly prednisone, are the primary pharmacological agents used in PMR management. The swift and substantial response to low to moderate corticosteroid doses is diagnostic and therapeutic.

> Tapering Schedule: The challenge lies in finding the balance between effective symptom control and minimizing the potential side effects of prolonged corticosteroid use. Healthcare professionals typically initiate treatment with a higher dose and gradually taper it as symptoms improve.

2. Disease-Modifying Antirheumatic Drugs (DMARDs):

> Methotrexate: In cases where corticosteroids alone are insufficient or when there is a need to minimize corticosteroid dosage, disease-modifying antirheumatic drugs (DMARDs) such as methotrexate may be considered as an adjunct therapy. Methotrexate is especially useful for individuals experiencing corticosteroid-related side effects.

3. Lifestyle Modifications:

Exercise and Physical Therapy: Regular physical activity, tailored to individual abilities, is crucial for maintaining joint flexibility and preventing muscle atrophy. Physical therapy may be recommended to address specific functional limitations and improve overall mobility.

Balanced Diet: While no specific PMR diet exists, adopting a balanced and nutritious diet is beneficial for overall health. Adequate calcium and vitamin D intake is essential to mitigate the bone-thinning effects of corticosteroids.

4. Monitoring and Follow-Up:

Regular Assessments: Ongoing monitoring is paramount to track disease activity, treatment response, and potential side effects of medications. Regular assessments allow for adjustments in treatment plans, including tapering corticosteroids when feasible.

Bone Health Monitoring: Given the increased risk of osteoporosis associated with long-term corticosteroid use, bone health assessments, including bone density scans, may be recommended.

5. Patient Education and Support:

Empowering Individuals: Providing comprehensive education about PMR, its treatment options, and potential side effects is vital for empowering individuals to participate actively in their care. Clear communication fosters informed decision-making and enhances adherence to treatment plans.

Support Groups: Connecting individuals with PMR to support groups or patient advocacy organizations can offer valuable emotional support, shared experiences, and practical tips for coping with the challenges of living with PMR.

6. Giant Cell Arteritis (GCA) Vigilance:

GCA Evaluation: As PMR and GCA often coexist, vigilant monitoring for symptoms of GCA, such as headaches, vision changes, and scalp tenderness, is essential. Timely diagnosis and intervention are critical to prevent complications associated with GCA.

CHAPTER TWO

The Role of Diet in Polymyalgia
Rheumatica (PMR)

Polymyalgia rheumatica (PMR), characterized by pain and stiffness in the shoulders, hips, and other areas, prompts a comprehensive approach to management. While medications play a central role, there is a growing recognition of the potential impact of diet on the inflammatory processes associated with PMR. This comprehensive overview explores the multifaceted role of diet in PMR, from influencing inflammation to supporting overall health and well-being.

1. Anti-Inflammatory Foods:

> Emphasis on Fruits and Vegetables: A diet rich in fruits and vegetables provides essential vitamins, minerals, and antioxidants with potential anti-inflammatory properties. These foods contribute to overall health and may help modulate the inflammatory response.

> Omega-3 Fatty Acids: Found in fatty fish, flaxseeds, chia seeds, and walnuts, omega-3 fatty acids exhibit anti-inflammatory effects. Including these sources in the diet may offer potential benefits for individuals with PMR.

2. Whole Grains and Legumes:

Complex Carbohydrates: Whole grains and legumes provide complex carbohydrates, fiber, and essential nutrients. These foods contribute to sustained energy levels, support digestive health, and may assist in maintaining a healthy weight.

Quinoa and Lentils: Quinoa and lentils, in particular, are excellent sources of protein and fiber, offering a nutrient-dense addition to a PMR-friendly diet.

3. Lean Proteins:

Poultry, Fish, and Plant-Based Proteins: Choosing lean protein sources such as poultry, fish, tofu, and legumes supports muscle health and provides essential amino acids. Plant-based proteins can be especially beneficial for those aiming to minimize the impact of animal fats on inflammation.

4. Limiting Inflammatory Triggers:

Processed Foods: Highly processed and refined foods often contain additives and preservatives that may contribute to inflammation. Minimizing the intake of processed foods and opting for whole, unprocessed options is advisable.

Limiting Sugar and Saturated Fats: Excessive consumption of sugar and saturated fats may promote inflammation. Monitoring the intake of sweets, sugary beverages, and high-fat foods supports an anti-inflammatory dietary approach.

5. Hydration:

Importance of Water: Staying well-hydrated is fundamental for overall health, and adequate water intake supports joint function, nutrient transport, and detoxification processes. Individuals with PMR are encouraged to prioritize water consumption throughout the day.

6. Potential Supplements:

Calcium and Vitamin D: Long-term corticosteroid use in PMR management may impact bone health. Adequate calcium and vitamin D intake through diet or supplements is essential to support bone density and mitigate the risk of osteoporosis.

Consultation with Healthcare Providers: Individuals should consult with their healthcare providers before incorporating supplements to ensure compatibility with their overall treatment plan and specific health needs.

7. Personalized Approach:

Consultation with Healthcare Professionals: The impact of diet on PMR varies among individuals, and dietary recommendations should be personalized. Consultation with healthcare professionals, including registered dietitians, can provide tailored guidance based on individual health status, preferences, and dietary restrictions.

BENEFITS OF FOLLOWING POLYMYALGIA RHEUMATICA DIET AS A POLYMYALGIA RHEUMATICA PATIENTS

Here are the Benefit Of Following Polymyalgia Rheumatica Diet As A Polymyalgia Rheumatica Patients:

1. Inflammation Management:

> Anti-Inflammatory Foods: A PMR-specific diet emphasizes the incorporation of anti-inflammatory foods such as fruits, vegetables, fatty fish, nuts, and seeds. These nutrient-rich choices have the potential to modulate the inflammatory processes associated with PMR, potentially leading to reduced pain and stiffness.

2. Supporting Joint Health:

Nutrient-Dense Choices: Nutrient-dense foods rich in vitamins, minerals, and antioxidants support joint health and function. Essential nutrients contribute to the repair and maintenance of connective tissues, potentially easing the impact of PMR on joints.

3. Weight Management:

Balanced Nutrition: Maintaining a healthy weight is crucial for individuals with PMR, as excess weight can exacerbate joint strain and inflammation. A PMR-specific diet, emphasizing whole foods and portion control, supports weight management and overall well-being.

4. Energy and Vitality:

Complex Carbohydrates: Whole grains and complex carbohydrates provide sustained energy, countering PMR fatigue. Including foods such as quinoa, brown rice, and legumes supports steady blood sugar levels and promotes vitality.

5. Bone Health:

Calcium and Vitamin D: Long-term corticosteroid use, a common treatment for PMR, can impact bone health. A diet rich in calcium and vitamin D, either through dietary choices or supplements, helps mitigate the risk of osteoporosis and supports overall bone density.

6. Gastrointestinal Health:

Fiber-Rich Foods: Including fiber-rich foods such as fruits, vegetables, and whole grains supports digestive health. Fiber contributes to regular bowel movements, potentially addressing gastrointestinal symptoms that some individuals with PMR may experience.

7. Psychological Well-being:

Mindful Eating: Adopting a PMR-specific diet fosters a sense of control and empowerment over one's health. Mindful eating and focusing on nutrient-dense choices positively impact mental well-being, offering a holistic approach to managing PMR.

8. Collaboration with Healthcare Providers:

Informed Decision-Making: Following a PMR-specific diet involves collaboration with healthcare providers, including rheumatologists and registered dietitians. Informed decision-making, based on individual health needs and treatment plans, ensures a comprehensive and tailored approach to dietary choices.

9. Community and Support:

Connecting with Others: Adopting a PMR-specific diet provides an opportunity for individuals to join with others facing similar challenges. Sharing experiences, recipe ideas, and practical tips through community and support groups can enhance the overall journey of managing PMR.

SAMPLE MEAL PLAN

Here is the sample meal plan for seven days for Polymyalgia Rheumatica Patients:

Day 1: Breakfast:

• Greek Yogurt Parfait with Mixed Berries and a Sprinkle of Chia Seeds

• Whole Grain Toast with Avocado

Lunch:

• Quinoa Salad with Chickpeas, Cucumber, Cherry Tomatoes, and Feta Cheese

• Lemon-Tahini Dressing

Snack:

• Fresh Apple Slices with Almond Butter

Dinner:

• Baked Salmon with a Herb and Lemon Marinade

• Roasted Sweet Potatoes

• Steamed Broccoli

Day 2: Breakfast:

• Spinach and Feta Omelette

• Whole Grain English Muffin

Lunch:

• Lentil and Vegetable Soup

• Whole Wheat Pita Bread

Snack:

• Carrot Sticks with Hummus

Dinner:

• Grilled Chicken Breast

• Quinoa Pilaf with Mixed Vegetables

• Sauteed Kale

Day 3: Breakfast:

• Smoothie Bowl with Spinach, Banana, Berries, and a Drizzle of Honey

• Topped with Granola and Pumpkin Seeds

Lunch:

• Whole Wheat Wrap with Turkey, Avocado, Spinach, and Dijon Mustard

• Side of Mixed Greens

Snack:

• Handful of Mixed Nuts (Walnuts, Almonds, and Pistachios)

Dinner:

• Stir-fried tofu with Broccoli, Bell Peppers, and Snow Peas

• Brown Rice

Day 4: Breakfast:

• Overnight Oats with Almond Milk, Chia Seeds, and Sliced Banana

Lunch:

- Quinoa and Black Bean Bowl with Corn, Avocado, and a Squeeze of Lime
- Fresh Cilantro Garnish

Snack:

- Greek Yogurt with a Drizzle of Honey

Dinner:

- Baked Cod with a Lemon-Herb Crust
- Roasted Brussels Sprouts
- Quinoa Salad with Cherry Tomatoes and Cucumber

Day 5: Breakfast:

- Whole Grain Pancakes with Fresh Berries and a Dollop of Greek Yogurt

Lunch:

- Chickpea and Vegetable Stir-Fry with Brown Rice
- Teriyaki Sauce

Snack:

- Sliced Mango with a Sprinkle of Tajin

Dinner:

- Grilled Shrimp Skewers with a Garlic-Lemon Marinade
- Quinoa Pilaf with Roasted Vegetables
- Steamed Asparagus

Day 6: Breakfast:

- Scrambled Eggs with Spinach and Feta
- Whole Grain Toast

Lunch:

• Mediterranean Chickpea Salad with Feta Cheese, Kalamata Olives, and Cherry Tomatoes

• Lemon-Olive Oil Dressing

Snack:

• Cottage Cheese with Pineapple Chunks

Dinner:

• Turkey and Quinoa Stuffed Bell Peppers

• Mixed Green Salad with Balsamic Vinaigrette

Day 7: Breakfast:

• Whole Grain Bagel with Smoked Salmon, Cream Cheese, and Capers

Lunch:

• Barley and Vegetable Stir-Fry with Tofu

• Soy-Ginger Sauce

Snack:

• Blueberry and Almond Smoothie

Dinner:

• Grilled Vegetable and Quinoa Bowl with a Green Tea-Infused Dressing

• Grilled Chicken Breast

SHOPPING LIST

Creating a thoughtful grocery shopping list is essential in adopting a diet that complements the management of Polymyalgia Rheumatica (PMR). This list encompasses a variety of nutrient-dense, anti-inflammatory foods to promote overall health and alleviate PMR symptoms. Adapt the quantities based on your preferences, dietary restrictions, and individual needs.

1. Fresh Produce:

> Leafy Greens: Spinach, kale, arugula

> Colorful Vegetables: Bell peppers, broccoli, Brussels sprouts, asparagus, cauliflower

> Berries: Blueberries, strawberries, raspberries

> Citrus Fruits: Oranges, lemons, limes

> Avocado

> Tomatoes

> Cucumber

> Fresh Herbs: Parsley, cilantro, mint

2. Whole Grains:

> Quinoa

> Brown Rice

> Whole Wheat Bread or Wraps

Oats

Barley

Whole Grain Pasta

3. Lean Proteins:

Salmon

Chicken Breast

Turkey

Tofu

Shrimp

Eggs

Greek Yogurt

4. Legumes:

Chickpeas

Lentils

Black Beans

5. Nuts and Seeds:

Almonds

Walnuts

Chia Seeds

Flaxseeds

Pumpkin Seeds

6. Dairy or Dairy Alternatives:

Greek Yogurt

Almond Milk or Other Non-Dairy Alternatives

Feta Cheese

7. Healthy Fats:

    Avocado Oil

    Olive Oil

8. Herbs and Spices:

    Turmeric

    Ginger

    Garlic

    Cumin

    Coriander

    Basil

    Cayenne Pepper

    Tajin (for seasoning fruits)

9. Frozen Foods:

    Wild-caught Fish Fillets (e.g., Cod)

    Mixed Berries

10. Canned Goods:

    Canned Tomatoes

    Canned Chickpeas

    Low-sodium chicken or Vegetable Broth

11. Condiments and Sauces:

    Dijon Mustard

    Soy Sauce (low-sodium)

    Tahini

    Lemon and Lime Juice

    Balsamic Vinegar

12. Sweeteners:

     Honey

     Maple Syrup

13. Grains and Legume Alternatives:

     Quinoa and Lentil Pastas

     Cauliflower Rice

14. Miscellaneous:

     Whole Grain Crackers

     Cottage Cheese

     Humus

     Green Tea Bags

CHAPTER THREE

Anti-Inflammatory Foods Recipes

Salmon and Berry Salad

Meal Description: This delightful Salmon and Berry Salad perfectly combines grilled salmon's savory richness and the refreshing burst of mixed berries. The vibrant mix of leafy greens provides a crisp backdrop, all brought together with a zesty citrus vinaigrette. This low-calorie, high-flavor dish is a celebration of wholesome ingredients and culinary balance.

Ingredients: For the Salad:

• Two salmon fillets (about 6 oz each)

• 4 cups mixed berries (strawberries, blueberries, raspberries)

• 6 cups mixed leafy greens (spinach, arugula, and watercress)

For the Citrus Vinaigrette:

• 1/4 cup extra-virgin olive oil

• Two tablespoons of fresh orange juice

• One tablespoon of fresh lemon juice

• One teaspoon of Dijon mustard

• One teaspoon honey

• Salt and pepper to taste

Instructions:

1. Grilling the Salmon:

• Preheat your grill or grill pan to medium-high heat.

• Season the salmon fillets with salt and pepper.

- Grill the salmon for about 4-5 minutes per side or until the internal temperature reaches 145°F (63°C), and the fish flakes easily with a fork.

2. Preparing the Berries and Greens:

- Wash and hull the berries as needed.

- In a large salad bowl, combine the mixed berries and leafy greens.

3. Making the Citrus Vinaigrette:

- Whisk together the olive oil, orange juice, lemon juice, Dijon mustard, honey, salt, and pepper in a small bowl until well combined.

4. Assembling the Salad:

- Place the grilled salmon fillets on top of the mixed berries and greens.

5. Drizzling with Citrus Vinaigrette:

- Drizzle the citrus vinaigrette over the entire salad just before serving.

6. Serving:

- Gently toss the salad to combine the flavors.

- Serve immediately, enjoying the contrast of warm grilled salmon with the excellent, crisp salad.

Nutrition Information (per serving):

- Calories: 240

- Protein: 24g

- Carbohydrates: 15g

- Fat: 10g

- Fiber: 5g

- Sugar: 8g
- Sodium: 80mg

TURMERIC CHICKPEA STEW

Meal Description: Indulge in the warmth and nourishment of our Turmeric Chickpea Stew. This hearty dish features chickpeas simmered to perfection with the vibrant duo of turmeric and ginger alongside an array of colorful vegetables, all bathed in a flavorful broth. Packed with wholesome goodness, this stew is a celebration of comforting flavors and healthful ingredients.

Ingredients: For the Stew:

• Two cans (15 oz each) of chickpeas, drained and rinsed

• One tablespoon of olive oil

• One onion, finely chopped

• Three cloves garlic, minced

• One tablespoon of fresh ginger, grated

• One teaspoon of ground turmeric

• One teaspoon of ground cumin

• One teaspoon of ground coriander

• 4 cups mixed vegetables (carrots, bell peppers, zucchini), diced

• One can (14 oz) diced tomatoes, undrained

• 4 cups vegetable broth

- Salt and pepper to taste

Optional Garnishes:

- Fresh cilantro, chopped

- Lemon wedges

Instructions:

1. Sautéing Aromatics:

- In a large pot, heat olive oil over medium heat.

- Add chopped onion, minced garlic, and grated ginger. Sauté until onions are translucent.

2. Adding Spices:

- Stir in ground turmeric, ground cumin, and ground coriander. Cook for an additional 1-2 minutes, making the spices fragrant.

3. Incorporating Chickpeas and Vegetables:

- Add chickpeas, diced mixed vegetables, diced tomatoes (with their juice), and vegetable broth to the pot.

- Season with salt and pepper to taste.

4. Simmering:

- Bring the stew to a boil, then reduce the heat to low. Cover and let it simmer for 20-25 minutes or until the vegetables are tender.

5. Adjusting Seasoning:

- Taste the stew and adjust the seasoning as needed. Add more salt, pepper, or spices according to your preference.

6. Serving:

- Ladle the Turmeric Chickpea Stew into bowls.

- Garnish with chopped fresh cilantro and serve with

lemon wedges on the side for an extra flavor.

7. Enjoying:

• Serve the stew hot, relishing the harmonious turmeric, ginger, and vegetable blend.

Nutrition Information (per serving):

• Calories: 280

• Protein: 10g

• Carbohydrates: 45g

• Fat: 7g

• Fiber: 12g

• Sugar: 8g

• Sodium: 800mg

AVOCADO AND SPINACH SMOOTHIE

Smoothie Description: Experience the rejuvenating power of our Avocado and Spinach Smoothie. This nutritious blend combines avocado's creamy richness with spinach's vibrant green goodness, enhanced by the sweetness of berries and the silky touch of almond milk. This smoothie is packed with essential nutrients and a delicious way to kickstart your day or replenish your energy.

Ingredients:

• One ripe avocado, peeled and pitted

• 2 cups fresh spinach leaves, washed

• 1 cup mixed berries (strawberries, blueberries, raspberries)

• 1 cup unsweetened almond milk

• Ice cubes (optional)

Instructions:

1. Preparing Ingredients:

• Cut the ripe avocado into chunks.

2. Blending:

• Combine the avocado chunks, fresh spinach leaves, mixed berries, and almond milk in a blender.

• You can add a handful of ice cubes if you prefer a colder smoothie.

3. Blending to Smooth Consistency:

• Blend the ingredients until the mixture reaches a smooth and creamy consistency.

4. Adjusting Consistency:

• If the smoothie is too thick, you can add more almond milk, a splash at a time, until it reaches your desired consistency.

5. Tasting and Adjusting:

• Add more berries or almond milk to taste the smoothie and adjust the sweetness or thickness.

6. Serving:

• Pour the Avocado and Spinach Smoothie into glasses.

7. Optional Garnish:

• Garnish with a few whole berries or a slice of avocado for a decorative touch.

8. Enjoying:

• Sip and savor this green elixir of vitality, reveling in the nourishing blend of avocado, spinach, berries, and almond milk.

Nutrition Information (per serving):

• Calories: 250

• Protein: 5g

• Carbohydrates: 25g

• Fat: 15g

• Fiber: 10g

- Sugar: 10g
- Sodium: 150mg

QUINOA AND ROASTED VEGETABLE BOWL

Bowl Description: Delight in the flavors and textures of our Quinoa and Roasted Vegetable Bowl, a vibrant dish that marries the wholesome goodness of quinoa with the robust taste of roasted bell peppers, zucchini, and cherry tomatoes. This nutritious bowl offers a satisfying medium of textures and colors, creating a feast for the eyes and palate.

Ingredients: For the Roasted Vegetables:

• One red bell pepper, sliced

• One yellow bell pepper, sliced

• One zucchini, sliced

• 1 cup cherry tomatoes, halved

• Two tablespoons of olive oil

• Salt and pepper to taste

• One teaspoon of dried oregano (optional)

For the Quinoa:

• 1 cup quinoa, rinsed

• 2 cups water or vegetable broth

• Salt to taste

Optional Garnish:

• Fresh basil or parsley, chopped

• Feta cheese, crumbled

Instructions:

1. Preparing the Quinoa:

• Rinse the quinoa under cold water.

• Combine the quinoa, water or vegetable broth, and a pinch of salt in a medium saucepan. Bring to a boil, then reduce the heat to low, cover, and simmer for 15-20 minutes or until the quinoa is cooked and the liquid is absorbed.

2. Preparing the Roasted Vegetables:

• Preheat the oven to 425°F (220°C).

• In a large bowl, toss the sliced bell peppers, zucchini, and halved cherry tomatoes with olive oil, salt, pepper, and dried oregano if using.

• Spread the vegetables on a baking sheet in a single layer.

• Roast in the oven for 20-25 minutes or until the vegetables are tender and slightly caramelized, stirring halfway through.

3. Assembling the Bowl:

• Spoon the cooked quinoa into serving bowls.

• Top with the roasted vegetables.

4. Optional Garnish:

• Garnish with fresh chopped basil or parsley and crumbled feta cheese for added flavor and freshness.

5. Enjoying:

• Toss the quinoa and roasted vegetables together before enjoying this colorful and nutritious bowl.

Nutrition Information (per serving):

• Calories: 350

• Protein: 10g

• Carbohydrates: 55g

• Fat: 10g

• Fiber: 8g

• Sugar: 5g

• Sodium: 300mg

GREEN TEA INFUSED QUINOA SALAD

Salad Description: Embark on a journey of freshness with our Green Tea Infused Quinoa Salad. This wholesome blend features the nutty richness of quinoa, crisp cucumber, and refreshing mint, all harmonized by a light and aromatic green tea-infused dressing. This salad not only tantalizes the taste buds but also provides a sense of tranquility in every bite.

Ingredients: For the Quinoa Salad:

- 1 cup quinoa, rinsed

- 2 cups water

- One cucumber, diced

- 1/4 cup fresh mint leaves, finely chopped

For the Green Tea Dressing:

- One green tea bag

- 1/4 cup hot water

- Two tablespoons of olive oil

- One tablespoon of rice vinegar

- One tablespoon of honey or maple syrup

- Salt and pepper to taste

Instructions:

1. Cooking the Quinoa:

• In a medium saucepan, combine the quinoa and water. Bring to a boil, then reduce the heat to low, cover, and simmer for 15-20 minutes or until the quinoa is cooked and the liquid is absorbed.

2. Brewing the Green Tea:

• Steep the green tea bag in hot water for 3-5 minutes. Allow it to cool.

3. Preparing the Green Tea Dressing:

• Combine the brewed green tea, olive oil, rice vinegar, honey or maple syrup, salt, and pepper in a small bowl. Whisk until well combined.

4. Assembling the Quinoa Salad:

• Combine the cooked quinoa, diced cucumber, and chopped fresh mint in a large bowl.

5. Infusing with Green Tea Dressing:

• Pour the green tea dressing over the quinoa salad.

• Gently toss the salad to ensure it is even coated with the dressing.

6. Chilling (Optional):

• Refrigerate the salad for 30 minutes to allow the flavors to meld, or serve immediately.

7. Serving:

• Spoon the Green Tea Infused Quinoa Salad onto plates or into bowls.

8. Enjoying:

• Savor each bite of this Zen Garden Medley, appreciating the delightful combination of quinoa, cucumber, mint, and the soothing essence of green tea.

Nutrition Information (per serving):

• Calories: 280

• Protein: 7g

• Carbohydrates: 45g

• Fat: 9g

• Fiber: 5g

• Sugar: 5g

• Sodium: 20mg

WALNUT-CRUSTED CHICKEN

Chicken Description: Elevate your chicken dinner with our Walnut-Crusted Chicken, a culinary masterpiece featuring succulent chicken breasts coated in a crunchy layer of crushed walnuts. Baked to perfection, this dish offers a harmonious blend of tender poultry and walnuts' rich, earthy essence. Prepare to embark on a journey of taste and texture with every delightful bite.

Ingredients:

• Four boneless, skinless chicken breasts

• 1 cup walnuts, finely chopped

• 1/2 cup breadcrumbs

• One teaspoon of dried thyme

• One teaspoon of garlic powder

• Salt and pepper to taste

• Two eggs, beaten

• Olive oil for drizzling

Instructions:

1. Preparing the Walnut Coating:

• Combine finely chopped walnuts, breadcrumbs, dried thyme, garlic powder, salt, and pepper in a shallow dish.

Mix well.

2. Preparing the Chicken:

• Preheat the oven to 375°F (190°C).

• Pat the chicken breasts dry with paper towels.

• Dip each chicken breast into the beaten eggs, ensuring an even coating.

3. Coating with Walnut Mixture:

• Roll the egg-coated chicken breasts in the walnut mixture, pressing gently to adhere the coating to all sides.

4. Placing on Baking Sheet:

• Place the walnut-crusted chicken breasts on a baking sheet lined with parchment paper.

5. Drizzling with Olive Oil:

• Drizzle a bit of olive oil over the top of each walnut-crusted chicken breast. This helps to enhance the crispiness of the coating.

6. Baking:

• Bake in the preheated oven for 20-25 minutes or until the internal temperature reaches 165°F (74°C) and the walnut crust is golden brown.

7. Resting and Slicing:

• Allow the ChickenChicken to rest for a few minutes before slicing. This helps to retain the juices.

8. Serving:

• Serve the Walnut-Crusted Chicken slices on a platter.

9. Enjoying:

• Revel in this Walnut-Crusted Chicken's Chicken's

delightful crunch and rich flavor, a culinary triumph that will leave your taste buds singing.

Nutrition Information (per serving):

• Calories: 350

• Protein: 30g

• Carbohydrates: 10g

• Fat: 22g

• Fiber: 3g

• Sugar: 1g

• Sodium: 400mg

PINEAPPLE TURMERIC SMOOTHIE BOWL

Smoothie Bowl Description: Embark on a taste journey with our Pineapple Turmeric Smoothie Bowl, a harmonious blend of tropical sweetness and the warm, earthy notes of turmeric. This refreshing bowl features the smooth texture of Greek yogurt, the vibrant hues of pineapple, and a delightful crunch from chia seeds. Indulge in this bowl for a burst of flavor that transports you to a sunny paradise.

Ingredients: For the Smoothie Base:

• 2 cups frozen pineapple chunks

• One teaspoon of ground turmeric

• 1 cup Greek yogurt (plain or vanilla)

• 1/2 cup almond milk (or any milk of choice)

For Topping:

• Chia seeds

• Additional pineapple chunks

Instructions:

1. Blending the Smoothie Base:

• Combine frozen pineapple chunks, ground turmeric, Greek yogurt, and almond milk in a blender.

• Blend until smooth and creamy. Add more almond milk if needed to reach your desired consistency.

2. Pouring into a Bowl:

• Pour the pineapple turmeric smoothie into a bowl.

3. Topping with Chia Seeds and Pineapple:

• Sprinkle chia seeds generously over the smoothie surface.

• Add additional pineapple chunks for a burst of freshness and texture.

4. Optional Garnish:

• You can drizzle a little honey over the top for an extra touch if desired.

5. Enjoying:

• Dive into this Tropical Sunrise Bliss with a spoon, savoring the combination of pineapple, turmeric, and the creaminess of Greek yogurt. Enjoy the satisfying crunch from chia seeds.

Nutrition Information (per serving):

• Calories: 300

• Protein: 15g

• Carbohydrates: 45g

• Fat: 7g

• Fiber: 8g

• Sugar: 30g

• Sodium: 80mg

MIXED BERRY CHIA PUDDING

Chia Pudding Description: Indulge in the richness of our Mixed Berry Chia Pudding, a delightful treat that combines the velvety smoothness of almond milk with the wholesome goodness of chia seeds. Topped with a vibrant mix of fresh berries, this pudding is visually appealing and has a burst of flavors and textures that will leave you craving more.

Ingredients: For the Chia Pudding:

• 1/4 cup chia seeds

• 1 cup almond milk (unsweetened)

• One tablespoon of maple syrup or honey (optional for sweetness)

• 1/2 teaspoon vanilla extract

For Topping:

• 1 cup mixed berries (strawberries, blueberries, raspberries)

• Fresh mint leaves for garnish (optional)

Instructions:

1. Mixing the Chia Pudding:

• In a bowl or jar, combine chia seeds, almond milk, maple

syrup (if using), and vanilla extract.

• Whisk the ingredients together until well combined.

2. Refrigerating the Mixture:

• Cover the bowl or jar and refrigerate for at least 2 hours or overnight, allowing the chia seeds to absorb the liquid and create a pudding-like consistency. Stir once or twice within the first hour to prevent clumping.

3. Topping with Berries:

• Spoon the chia pudding into serving bowls or glasses once the chia pudding has been set.

• Top generously with a mix of fresh berries.

4. Garnishing (Optional):

• Garnish with fresh mint leaves for a touch of freshness.

5. Serving:

• Serve chilled, and enjoy the Mixed Berry Chia Pudding with a spoon.

6. Savoring:

• Revel in the delightful contrast of the smooth chia pudding against the burst of flavor from the mixed berries.

Nutrition Information (per serving):

• Calories: 200

• Protein: 6g

• Carbohydrates: 25g

• Fat: 9g

• Fiber: 12g

• Sugar: 10g

- Sodium: 100mg

CHAPTER FOUR

Omega-3 Fatty Acids Recipes

Grilled Mackerel Tacos

Taco Description: Transport your taste buds to the seaside with our Grilled Mackerel Tacos—a celebration of tender mackerel fillets, kissed by the grill and enveloped in whole grain tortillas. Crowned with a zesty cabbage slaw, these tacos promise a burst of oceanic flavors in every bite. Get ready for a fiesta of freshness and savory delights.

Ingredients: For the Grilled Mackerel:

- Four mackerel fillets

- Two tablespoons of olive oil

- One teaspoon of smoked paprika

- One teaspoon of ground cumin

- Salt and pepper to taste

- Lime wedges for serving

For the Cabbage Slaw:

- 2 cups shredded green cabbage

- One carrot, julienned

- 1/4 cup fresh cilantro, chopped

- Two tablespoons mayonnaise

- One tablespoon of lime juice

- Salt and pepper to taste

For Assembling Tacos:

- Whole grain tortillas

- Avocado slices (optional)

Instructions:

1. Preparing the Grilled Mackerel:

• Preheat the grill to medium-high heat.

• Mix olive oil, smoked paprika, ground cumin, salt, and pepper in a bowl.

• Brush the mackerel fillets with the spice mixture.

2. Grilling the Mackerel:

• Grill the mackerel fillets for 3-4 minutes per side or until cooked through and grill marks appear.

• Remove from the grill and squeeze fresh lime juice over the fillets.

3. Making the Cabbage Slaw:

• Combine shredded cabbage, julienned carrot, chopped cilantro, mayonnaise, lime juice, salt, and pepper in a separate bowl. Toss until well coated.

4. Assembling the Tacos:

• Heat the whole-grain tortillas according to package instructions.

• Place a grilled mackerel fillet in each tortilla.

• Top with a generous portion of cabbage slaw.

5. Optional Garnish:

• Garnish with avocado slices for an extra creamy touch.

6. Serving:

• Serve the Grilled Mackerel Tacos hot, ready for a flavor fiesta.

7. Enjoying:

• Sink your teeth into the oceanic delights of these tacos, savoring the perfect harmony of grilled mackerel and zesty cabbage slaw.

Nutrition Information (per serving):

- Calories: 350
- Protein: 25g
- Carbohydrates: 20g
- Fat: 20g
- Fiber: 5g
- Sugar: 3g
- Sodium: 400mg

FLAXSEED-CRUSTED BAKED COD

Cod Description: Elevate your seafood experience with our Flaxseed-Crusted Baked Cod—a culinary masterpiece that combines the delicate flakiness of cod with the nutty crunch of ground flaxseeds. Baked to golden perfection, these fillets promise a flavorful journey that's delicious and packed with wholesome goodness.

Ingredients: For the Flaxseed Crust:

• Four cod fillets

• 1 cup ground flaxseeds

• One teaspoon of garlic powder

• One teaspoon paprika

• Salt and pepper to taste

• Two tablespoons Dijon mustard (for coating)

For Serving:

• Lemon wedges

• Fresh parsley, chopped (optional)

Instructions:

1. Preparing the Flaxseed Crust:

• Preheat the oven to 400°F (200°C).

• Mix ground flaxseeds, garlic powder, paprika, salt, and pepper in a shallow bowl.

2. Coating the Cod:

• Pat the cod fillets dry with paper towels.

• Brush each fillet with a thin layer of Dijon mustard.

3. Dredging in Flaxseed Mixture:

• Dip each cod fillet into the flaxseed mixture, pressing the mixture onto the fillets to coat them evenly.

4. Placing on Baking Sheet:

• Place the coated cod fillets on a baking sheet lined with parchment paper.

5. Baking:

• Bake in the preheated oven for 12-15 minutes or until the cod is cooked through and the flaxseed crust is crispy and golden.

6. Serving:

• Carefully transfer the Flaxseed-Crusted Baked Cod to serving plates.

7. Garnishing:

• Squeeze fresh lemon juice over the cod fillets.

• Garnish with chopped fresh parsley if desired.

8. Enjoying:

• Delight in the exquisite combination of flaky cod and the nutty crunch of the flaxseed crust. Serve with additional lemon wedges on the side.

Nutrition Information (per serving):

• Calories: 250

- Protein: 30g
- Carbohydrates: 10g
- Fat: 12g
- Fiber: 8g
- Sugar: 1g
- Sodium: 350mg

CHIA SEED AND BERRY POPSICLES

Popsicle Description: Beat the heat with our Chia Seed and Berry Popsicles—a delightful fusion of nutrient-packed chia seeds, hydrating coconut water, and a burst of mixed berries. These frozen treats offer a refreshing respite and bring together the goodness of chia and the vibrant flavors of summer berries in every incredible bite.

Ingredients:

- 1/4 cup chia seeds

- 1 cup coconut water

- Two tablespoons honey or agave syrup (optional for sweetness)

- 1 cup mixed berries (strawberries, blueberries, raspberries)

- Popsicle molds and sticks

Instructions:

1. Preparing the Chia Seed Mixture:

- In a bowl, combine chia seeds, coconut water, and honey or agave syrup (if using).

- Stir well and let it sit for 10-15 minutes until the chia seeds absorb the liquid and form a gel-like consistency.

2. Blending the Berry Mixture:

• Combine mixed berries in a blender until you achieve a smooth puree.

3. Layering the Popsicles:

• In the popsicle molds, alternately layer the chia seed mixture and berry puree.

• Use a spoon to mix the layers gently for a marbled effect.

4. Inserting Sticks:

• Place the popsicle sticks into the molds.

5. Freezing:

• Freeze the popsicles for at least 4-6 hours or until they are completely set.

6. Unmolding:

• Once fully frozen, run the popsicle molds under warm water for a few seconds to help release the popsicles.

7. Serving:

• Serve the Chia Seed and Berry Popsicles immediately for a refreshing treat.

8. Enjoying:

• Cool down and savor the delightful combination of chia seeds and summer berries in these Berrylicious Cool Bites.

Note:

• Feel free to customize the sweetness of the popsicles by adjusting the amount of honey or agave syrup.

• You can also add a squeeze of lime juice to the berry puree for an extra zesty kick.

Nutrition Information (per popsicle):

- Calories: 80
- Protein: 2g
- Carbohydrates: 12g
- Fat: 3g
- Fiber: 5g
- Sugar: 5g
- Sodium: 10mg

SALMON AND AVOCADO SUSHI BOWLS

Bowl Description: Experience the flavors of sushi in a simplified and satisfying form with our Salmon and Avocado Sushi Bowls. These bowls feature a bed of seasoned sushi rice adorned with grilled salmon, creamy avocado slices, and the umami richness of seaweed strips. Get ready to indulge in a delicious and easy-to-assemble, deconstructed sushi masterpiece.

Ingredients: For the Sushi Rice:

• 2 cups sushi rice

• 1/3 cup rice vinegar

• Two tablespoons sugar

• One teaspoon salt

For the Bowl:

• Four salmon fillets, grilled or pan-seared

• Two ripe avocados, sliced

• Seaweed strips or nori, cut into thin strips

• Soy sauce for drizzling

• Pickled ginger and wasabi (optional for serving)

Instructions:

1. Cooking the Sushi Rice:

• Rinse the sushi rice under cold water until the water runs clear.

• Cook the rice according to package instructions.

• Heat the rice vinegar, sugar, and salt in a small saucepan until the sugar and salt dissolve. Let it cool.

• Once the rice is cooked, transfer it to a large bowl and gently fold in the vinegar mixture. Allow it to cool to room temperature.

2. Grilling the Salmon:

• Grill or pan-sear the salmon fillets until cooked through, approximately 3-4 minutes per side, or to your desired level of doneness.

3. Assembling the Bowls:

• Divide the sushi rice among serving bowls.

• Top each bowl with a grilled salmon fillet, sliced avocado, and seaweed strips.

4. Drizzling with Soy Sauce:

• Drizzle a bit of soy sauce over the salmon and avocado.

5. Optional Garnishes:

• Serve the Salmon and Avocado Sushi Bowls with pickled ginger, wasabi, and additional soy sauce on the side.

6. Enjoying:

• Dive into these delectable sushi bowls, relishing the combination of tender grilled salmon, creamy avocado, and the delightful contrast of sushi rice.

Note:

• Feel free to customize your bowls with additional toppings such as cucumber, sesame seeds, or radishes for added crunch and flavor.

Nutrition Information (per serving):

• Calories: 500

• Protein: 30g

• Carbohydrates: 60g

• Fat: 18g

• Fiber: 5g

• Sugar: 1g

• Sodium: 800mg

HEMP SEED AND BANANA SMOOTHIE

Smoothie Description: Revitalize your day with our Hemp Seed and Banana Smoothie. This nourishing blend combines the nutty goodness of hemp seeds with the natural sweetness of ripe banana; all enveloped in the smooth embrace of almond milk. Packed with protein and essential nutrients, this smoothie is delicious and a wholesome elixir to fuel your day.

Ingredients:

• Two tablespoons hemp seeds

• One ripe banana

• 1 cup almond milk (unsweetened)

• Ice cubes (optional)

Instructions:

1. Preparing the Ingredients:

• Peel the ripe banana and break it into chunks.

2. Blending:

• Combine the hemp seeds, banana chunks, and almond milk in a blender.

• You can add a handful of ice cubes if you prefer a colder smoothie.

3. Blending to Smooth Consistency:

• Blend the ingredients until the mixture reaches a smooth and creamy consistency.

4. Adjusting Consistency:

• If the smoothie is too thick, you can add more almond milk, a splash at a time, until it reaches your desired consistency.

5. Tasting and Adjusting:

• Taste the smoothie and adjust the sweetness or thickness by adding more banana or almond milk if needed.

6. Serving:

• Pour the Hemp Seed and Banana Smoothie into glasses.

7. Enjoying:

• Sip and savor this nutrient-packed elixir, relishing the combination of hemp seeds, banana, and the creamy texture of almond milk.

Nutrition Information (per serving):

• Calories: 300

• Protein: 10g

• Carbohydrates: 30g

• Fat: 15g

• Fiber: 8g

• Sugar: 12g

• Sodium: 150mg

TUNA AND QUINOA STUFFED PEPPERS

Stuffed Pepper Description: Elevate your stuffed peppers game with our Tuna and Quinoa Stuffed Peppers—an enticing blend of protein-packed tuna and wholesome Quinoa combined with vibrant bell peppers and baked to perfection. These stuffed peppers offer a harmonious fusion of textures and flavors that will satisfy your taste buds and make you crave more.

Ingredients:

• Four bell peppers, halved and seeds removed

• 1 cup quinoa, cooked

• Two cans (5 oz each) of tuna, drained

• 1 cup cherry tomatoes, halved

• 1/2 cup red onion, finely diced

• 1/4 cup black olives, sliced

• Two cloves garlic, minced

• One teaspoon dried oregano

• One teaspoon of ground cumin

• Salt and pepper to taste

• 1 cup feta cheese, crumbled (optional for topping)

- Fresh parsley, chopped (for garnish)

Instructions:

1. Preparing the Bell Peppers:

- Preheat the oven to 375°F (190°C).

- Cut the bell peppers in half lengthwise, removing seeds and membranes.

2. Cooking Quinoa:

- Cook the Quinoa according to package instructions.

3. Preparing the Filling:

- Combine the cooked Quinoa, drained tuna, cherry tomatoes, red onion, black olives, minced garlic, dried oregano, ground cumin, salt, and pepper in a large bowl. Mix well.

4. Stuffing the Peppers:

- Place the bell pepper halves on a baking sheet.

- Generously stuff each pepper half with the tuna and quinoa mixture.

5. Baking:

- Bake in the preheated oven for 25-30 minutes or until the peppers are tender.

6. Optional Topping:

- If desired, sprinkle crumbled feta cheese over the stuffed peppers during the last 5 minutes of baking.

7. Garnishing:

- Remove the stuffed peppers from the oven and garnish with fresh chopped parsley.

8. Serving:

• Serve the Tuna and Quinoa Stuffed Peppers hot, allowing the flavors to meld.

9. Enjoying:

• Delight in the flavorful fusion of tuna, Quinoa, and Mediterranean-inspired ingredients in every bite.

Nutrition Information (per serving):

• Calories: 350

• Protein: 25g

• Carbohydrates: 35g

• Fat: 14g

• Fiber: 6g

• Sugar: 5g

• Sodium: 500mg

OMEGA-3 RICH TRAIL MIX

Trail Mix Description: Elevate your snack game with our Omega-3 Rich Trail Mix—a powerhouse combination of walnuts, almonds, chia seeds, and dried berries. Packed with omega-3 fatty acids, protein, and antioxidants, this trail mix not only satisfies your snack cravings but also provides a boost of energy and essential nutrients. Grab a handful and enjoy a tasty and nutritious pick-me-up!

Ingredients:

- 1 cup walnuts

- 1 cup almonds

- 1/4 cup chia seeds

- 1/2 cup dried blueberries

- 1/2 cup dried cranberries

- 1/4 cup dried goji berries

Instructions:

1. Selecting Quality Ingredients:

• Ensure that the nuts and seeds are fresh and of high quality.

2. Preparing the Nuts:

• If the walnuts and almonds are not already chopped, you

can roughly chop them to your desired size.

3. Combining Ingredients:

• In a large mixing bowl, combine the walnuts, almonds, chia seeds, dried blueberries, dried cranberries, and dried goji berries.

4. Tossing and Mixing:

• Toss the ingredients together until well mixed, ensuring an even distribution of nuts, seeds, and dried berries.

5. Portioning:

• Portion the trail mix into small, snack-sized containers or resealable bags for convenient grab-and-go snacks.

6. Storing:

• Store the Omega-3 Rich Trail Mix in an airtight container in a cool, dry place to maintain freshness.

7. Enjoying:

• Grab a handful of this nutrient-packed trail mix whenever you need a quick and healthy snack.

Note:

• Feel free to customize the trail mix by adding other favorite nuts, seeds, or dried fruits to suit your taste preferences.

• Consider portioning the trail mix into individual serving sizes to avoid overeating.

Nutrition Information (per serving - approximately 1/4 cup):

• Calories: 180

• Protein: 5g

- Carbohydrates: 15g
- Fat: 12g
- Fiber: 4g
- Sugar: 7g
- Sodium: 5mg

SARDINE AND OLIVE TAPENADE

Tapenade Description: Transport your taste buds to the Mediterranean with our Sardine and Olive Tapenade—a savory blend of sardines, olives, garlic, and olive oil. This flavorful tapenade, rich in omega-3 fatty acids, perfectly accompanies whole-grain crackers. Whether served as an appetizer or a snack, indulge in the robust flavors of the sea and the Mediterranean sun.

Ingredients:

• One can (4.4 oz) sardines in olive oil, drained

• 1 cup black olives, pitted

• Two cloves garlic, minced

• Two tablespoons of capers drained

• Two tablespoons fresh parsley, chopped

• Two tablespoons extra virgin olive oil

• Freshly ground black pepper, to taste

• Whole grain crackers for serving

Instructions:

1. Preparing the Ingredients:

• Ensure the sardines are drained of excess oil.

• Pit the black olives if they aren't already pitted.

• Mince the garlic cloves.

2. Blending the Tapenade:

• Combine the drained sardines, black olives, minced garlic, capers, and fresh parsley in a food processor.

• Pulse the ingredients until you achieve a coarse paste.

3. Drizzling Olive Oil:

• While the food processor is running, gradually drizzle in the extra virgin olive oil.

• Continue processing until the tapenade reaches your desired consistency.

4. Seasoning:

• Season the tapenade with freshly ground black pepper to taste. The olives and capers are naturally salty, so additional salt may not be necessary.

5. Serving:

• Spoon the Sardine and Olive tapenade into a serving bowl.

6. Accompanying with Crackers:

• Serve the tapenade with whole-grain crackers for a wholesome pairing.

7. Enjoying:

• Dive into the flavors of the Mediterranean with each bite of this Sardine and Olive Tapenade, reveling in the richness of sardines, the saltiness of olives, and the aromatic notes of garlic.

Note:

• Adjust the consistency by adding more olive oil if you

prefer a smoother texture.

• This tapenade can also be used as a spread on whole-grain bread or as a topping for grilled vegetables.

Nutrition Information (per serving - approximately two tablespoons):

• Calories: 80

• Protein: 4g

• Carbohydrates: 2g

• Fat: 7g

• Fiber: 1g

• Sugar: 0g

• Sodium: 200mg

CHAPTER FIVE

Whole Grains Recipes

Brown Rice and Lentil Soup

Soup Description: Warm your soul with our Brown Rice and Lentil Soup—a nourishing blend of wholesome brown rice, protein-packed lentils, and a medley of colorful vegetables. This hearty soup is delicious and a healthy and comforting meal that will satisfy you. Perfect for cozy evenings or whenever you need a bowl of hearty goodness.

Ingredients:

- 1 cup brown lentils, rinsed and drained

- 1 cup brown rice

- One tablespoon of olive oil

- One onion, finely chopped

- Two carrots diced

- Two celery stalks, diced

- Three cloves garlic, minced

- One teaspoon of ground cumin

- One teaspoon paprika

- 1/2 teaspoon ground coriander

- 1/2 teaspoon dried thyme

- 6 cups vegetable or chicken broth

- One can (14 oz) diced tomatoes, undrained

- Salt and pepper to taste

- Fresh parsley, chopped (for garnish)

Instructions:

1. Preparing Lentils and Rice:

• Rinse the brown lentils under cold water and drain.

• Rinse the brown rice under cold water.

2. Sautéing Aromatics:

• In a large pot, heat olive oil over medium heat.

• Add chopped onion, diced carrots, and diced celery. Sauté until vegetables are softened, about 5 minutes.

3. Adding Aromatics and Spices:

• Add minced garlic, ground cumin, paprika, ground coriander, and dried thyme. Stir to combine and cook for an additional 1-2 minutes until fragrant.

4. Cooking Lentils and Rice:

• Add the rinsed lentils, brown rice, vegetable or chicken broth, and diced tomatoes (with their juice) to the pot.

• Season with salt and pepper to taste.

5. Bringing to a Boil:

• Bring the soup to a boil, then reduce the heat to low, cover, and simmer for 40-45 minutes or until the lentils and rice are tender.

6. Adjusting Seasoning:

• Taste the soup and adjust the seasoning if needed. Add more salt and pepper according to your preference.

7. Serving:

• Ladle the Brown Rice and Lentil Soup into bowls.

8. Garnishing:

• Garnish with fresh chopped parsley.

9. Enjoying:

• Enjoy this hearty and nutritious soup, relishing the

combination of lentils, brown rice, and a medley of vegetables.

Note:

• You can customize the soup by adding additional vegetables such as spinach or kale.

• Consider drizzling each serving with a bit of olive oil for extra richness.

Nutrition Information (per serving):

• Calories: 300

• Protein: 12g

• Carbohydrates: 55g

• Fat: 4g

• Fiber: 10g

• Sugar: 5g

• Sodium: 800mg

QUINOA AND BLACK BEAN BURRITO BOWLS

Bowl Description: Experience a burst of Southwestern flavors with our Quinoa and Black Bean Burrito Bowls. These vibrant bowls showcase a hearty combination of protein-packed quinoa, savory black beans, sweet corn, creamy avocado, and a zesty squeeze of Lime. Each bite celebrates wholesome ingredients that come together in perfect harmony.

Ingredients:

• 1 cup quinoa, rinsed

• 2 cups black beans, cooked or canned (drained and rinsed)

• 1 cup corn kernels (fresh, frozen, or canned)

• One ripe avocado, sliced

• One lime, cut into wedges

• Fresh cilantro, chopped (for garnish)

• Salt and pepper to taste

• Optional toppings: salsa, shredded cheese, Greek yogurt

Instructions:

1. Cooking Quinoa:

• In a saucepan, combine the rinsed quinoa with 2 cups of water. Bring to a boil, then reduce the heat, cover, and simmer for 15-20 minutes or until the quinoa is cooked and water is absorbed.

2. Preparing Black Beans:

• If using canned black beans, drain and rinse them. If using cooked black beans, ensure they are warmed.

3. Cooking Corn:

• If using fresh or frozen corn, cook it according to package instructions. If using canned corn, drain it.

4. Assembling the Bowls:

• Divide the cooked quinoa, black beans, and corn among serving bowls.

5. Adding Avocado:

• Top each bowl with slices of ripe avocado.

6. Squeezing Lime:

• Squeeze fresh lime wedges over each bowl for a burst of citrusy freshness.

7. Seasoning:

• Season the bowls with salt and pepper to taste.

8. Garnishing:

• Garnish with chopped fresh cilantro.

9. Optional Toppings:

• Customize your bowls with optional toppings such as salsa, shredded cheese, or a dollop of Greek yogurt.

10. Enjoying:

• Dive into the Southwestern bliss of these Quinoa and

Black Bean Burrito Bowls, savoring the blend of textures and flavors in each spoonful.

Note:

• Feel free to add protein like grilled chicken, shrimp, or tofu for an extra boost.

• These bowls can be meal-prepped for quick and convenient lunches.

Nutrition Information (per serving):

• Calories: 400

• Protein: 15g

• Carbohydrates: 65g

• Fat: 12g

• Fiber: 15g

• Sugar: 3g

• Sodium: 300mg

WHOLE WHEAT PASTA PRIMAVERA

Pasta Description: Savor the wholesome goodness of our Whole Wheat Pasta Primavera—a delightful medley of colorful vegetables dancing on a bed of whole wheat pasta, embraced by a light and flavorful tomato sauce. This dish not only satisfies your pasta cravings but also brings the freshness of the garden to your plate. Prepare to indulge in a symphony of taste and texture!

Ingredients:

- 8 oz whole wheat pasta
- Two tablespoons of olive oil
- Three cloves garlic, minced
- One red bell pepper, thinly sliced
- One yellow bell pepper, thinly sliced
- 1 zucchini, julienned
- One carrot, julienned
- 1 cup cherry tomatoes, halved
- 1 cup broccoli florets, blanched
- 1/2 cup snap peas, trimmed
- One can (14 oz) crushed tomatoes

• One teaspoon dried oregano

• One teaspoon of dried basil

• Salt and pepper to taste

• Grated Parmesan cheese for serving

• Fresh basil, chopped (for garnish)

Instructions:

1. Cooking Whole Wheat Pasta:

• Cook the whole wheat pasta according to package instructions until al dente. Drain and set aside.

2. Sautéing Aromatics:

• In a large skillet, heat olive oil over medium heat. Add minced garlic and sauté for 1-2 minutes until fragrant.

3. Adding Vegetables:

• Add thinly sliced red and yellow bell peppers, julienned zucchini, and carrot to the skillet. Sauté until the vegetables are slightly tender, about 5 minutes.

4. Introducing Cherry Tomatoes and Greens:

• Add halved cherry tomatoes, blanched broccoli florets, and trimmed snap peas to the skillet. Cook for an additional 3-4 minutes.

5. Preparing Tomato Sauce:

• Pour in the crushed tomatoes and sprinkle with dried oregano, dried basil, salt, and pepper. Stir well to combine.

6. Simmering:

• Let the Sauce simmer for 10-15 minutes, allowing the flavors to meld and the vegetables to cook thoroughly.

7. Combining with Whole Wheat Pasta:

• Add the cooked whole wheat pasta to the skillet, tossing to coat the pasta evenly with the vegetable and tomato mixture.

8. Serving:

• Serve the Whole Wheat Pasta Primavera in bowls.

9. Garnishing:

• Garnish with grated Parmesan cheese and fresh chopped basil.

10. Enjoying:

• Enjoy this vibrant and wholesome pasta dish, reveling in the symphony of colors and flavors.

Note:

• Feel free to customize the vegetables based on your preferences and what's in season.

• You can incorporate grilled chicken, shrimp, or chickpeas for added protein.

Nutrition Information (per serving):

• Calories: 400

• Protein: 14g

• Carbohydrates: 70g

• Fat: 8g

• Fiber: 12g

• Sugar: 8g

• Sodium: 400mg

BARLEY AND VEGETABLE STIR-FRY

Stir-Fry Description: Elevate your stir-fry game with our Barley and Vegetable Stir-Fry—a wholesome fusion of chewy Barley, vibrant mixed vegetables, tofu, and a flavorful soy-ginger sauce. This dish not only tantalizes your taste buds with its medley of textures and tastes but also provides a nutritious and satisfying meal perfect for any day of the week.

Ingredients:

• 1 cup barley, cooked

• 1 cup firm tofu, cubed

• Two tablespoons of sesame oil

• 3 cups mixed vegetables (broccoli, bell peppers, snap peas, carrots), chopped

• Three cloves garlic, minced

• One tablespoon of fresh ginger, grated

• 1/4 cup low-sodium soy sauce

• One tablespoon of rice vinegar

• One tablespoon of honey or maple syrup

• One teaspoon of cornstarch (optional for thickening)

• Sesame seeds for garnish

• Green onions, chopped (for garnish)

Instructions:

1. Preparing Barley:

• Cook the Barley according to package instructions. Set aside.

2. Pan-Frying Tofu:

• Heat one tablespoon of sesame oil over medium-high heat in a large wok or skillet.

• Add cubed tofu and cook until golden brown on all sides. Remove tofu from the wok and set aside.

3. Sautéing Aromatics:

• In the same wok, add the remaining tablespoon of sesame oil.

• Add minced garlic and grated ginger, sautéing for about 1 minute until fragrant.

4. Stir-Frying Vegetables:

• Add the chopped mixed vegetables to the wok. Stir-fry until the vegetables are crisp-tender, about 5-7 minutes.

5. Preparing Soy-Ginger Sauce:

• Whisk together soy sauce, rice vinegar, and honey or maple syrup in a small bowl.

• If desired, mix in cornstarch to thicken the Sauce.

6. Combining Barley and Tofu:

• Add the cooked Barley and pan-fried tofu back to the wok.

7. Pouring Sauce:

• Pour the soy-ginger sauce over the Barley, tofu, and vegetables. Toss everything together until well coated.

8. Garnishing:

• Garnish the stir-fry with sesame seeds and chopped green onions.

9. Serving:

• Serve the Barley and Vegetable Stir-Fry hot, savoring the combination of textures and flavors.

10. Enjoying:

• Dive into this wholesome wok delight, relishing Barley's chewiness, the vegetables' crunch, and the soy-ginger sauce's savory notes.

Note:

• Feel free to customize the vegetables based on your preferences and what's in season.

• Adjust the sweetness and saltiness of the Sauce according to your taste.

Nutrition Information (per serving):

• Calories: 400

• Protein: 15g

• Carbohydrates: 60g

• Fat: 12g

• Fiber: 10g

• Sugar: 8g

• Sodium: 600mg

FARRO AND ROASTED VEGETABLE SALAD

Salad Description: Indulge in the essence of autumn with our Farro and Roasted Vegetable Salad—a hearty blend of nutty Farro, caramelized butternut squash, roasted Brussels sprouts, and a zesty lemon vinaigrette. This salad not only celebrates the robust flavors of the season but also delivers a satisfying and nutritious dish that's perfect as a wholesome lunch or a delightful side at dinner.

Ingredients:

For the Salad:

- 1 cup farro, rinsed

- 2 cups butternut squash, peeled and diced

- 2 cups Brussels sprouts, trimmed and halved

- Two tablespoons of olive oil

- Salt and pepper to taste

For the Lemon Vinaigrette:

- 1/4 cup extra virgin olive oil

- Zest and juice of 1 lemon

- One tablespoon of Dijon mustard

• One clove garlic, minced

• Salt and pepper to taste

Optional Garnish:

• Crumbled feta cheese

• Toasted pumpkin seeds

• Fresh parsley, chopped

Instructions:

1. Preparing Farro:

• Cook the Farro according to package instructions. Once cooked, drain any excess water and let it cool.

2. Roasting Vegetables:

• Preheat the oven to 400°F (200°C).

• Toss the diced butternut squash and halved Brussels sprouts on a baking sheet with olive oil, salt, and pepper.

• Roast in the preheated oven for 25-30 minutes or until the vegetables are tender and caramelized, stirring halfway through.

3. Preparing Lemon Vinaigrette:

• Whisk together extra virgin olive oil, lemon zest, lemon juice, Dijon mustard, minced garlic, salt, and pepper in a small bowl.

4. Assembling the Salad:

• Combine the cooked Farro, roasted butternut squash, and Brussels sprouts in a large bowl.

5. Dressing the Salad:

• Pour the lemon vinaigrette over the salad and toss gently to coat all the ingredients.

6. Optional Garnish:

• If desired, sprinkle crumbled feta cheese, toasted pumpkin seeds, and chopped fresh parsley over the salad.

7. Serving:

• Serve the Farro and Roasted Vegetable Salad at room temperature or chilled.

8. Enjoying:

• Savor the rich flavors and textures of this harvest-inspired salad, relishing the farro nuttiness, butternut squash sweetness, and the depth of roasted Brussels sprouts.

Note:

• Feel free to customize the salad with additional ingredients like dried cranberries or roasted pecans for extra sweetness and crunch.

• This salad can be made ahead of time and refrigerated. The flavors often develop even more when allowed to marinate.

Nutrition Information (per serving):

• Calories: 350

• Protein: 8g

• Carbohydrates: 55g

• Fat: 15g

• Fiber: 10g

• Sugar: 4g

• Sodium: 200mg

BUCKWHEAT PANCAKES WITH BERRIES

Pancake Description: Start your morning with our Buckwheat Pancakes—a stack of fluffy goodness made with nutty buckwheat flour and topped with fresh berries. This wholesome breakfast delights your taste buds and provides a nutritious and energizing way to kick off your day. Get ready to indulge in the perfect balance of hearty and sweet flavors.

Ingredients:

For the Pancakes:

• 1 cup buckwheat flour

• One tablespoon sugar

• One teaspoon baking powder

• 1/2 teaspoon baking soda

• 1/4 teaspoon salt

• 1 cup buttermilk

• One large egg

• Two tablespoons unsalted butter, melted

• Cooking spray or additional butter for greasing the skillet

For Topping:

• Fresh mixed berries (strawberries, blueberries, raspberries)

• Maple syrup (optional)

Instructions:

1. Preparing the Batter:

• Whisk together buckwheat flour, sugar, baking powder, baking soda, and salt in a large bowl.

2. Mixing Wet Ingredients:

• Whisk together buttermilk, egg, and melted butter in a separate bowl.

3. Combining Wet and Dry Ingredients:

• Pour the wet ingredients into the dry ingredients and gently stir until combined. Do not overmix; a few lumps are okay.

4. Resting the Batter:

• Let the batter rest for 10-15 minutes, allowing the buckwheat flour to absorb the liquid.

5. Preheating the Griddle:

• Preheat a grill or non-stick skillet over medium heat. Lightly grease with cooking spray or butter.

6. Cooking the Pancakes:

• Pour 1/4 cup of batter onto the hot griddle for each pancake. Cook until bubbles form on the surface, then flip and cook the other side until golden brown.

7. Keeping Warm:

• Keep the cooked pancakes warm in a low oven (about

200°F or 93°C) while you cook the remaining batter.

8. Topping with Berries:

• Stack the pancakes on a plate and top with a generous amount of fresh mixed berries.

9. Optional Maple Syrup:

• Drizzle with maple syrup if desired.

10. Enjoying:

• Dive into these Buckwheat Pancakes with Berries, savoring the hearty flavor of buckwheat and the natural sweetness of fresh berries.

Note:

• Buckwheat flour can sometimes be dense, but these pancakes are light and fluffy due to the combination of buttermilk and baking powder.

• Feel free to customize the topping with a dollop of Greek yogurt or a sprinkle of chopped nuts.

Nutrition Information (per serving - 2 pancakes):

• Calories: 250

• Protein: 7g

• Carbohydrates: 35g

• Fat: 9g

• Fiber: 5g

• Sugar: 5g

• Sodium: 400mg

CAULIFLOWER FRIED RICE WITH QUINOA

Fried Rice Description: Experience the savory satisfaction of our Cauliflower Fried Rice with Quinoa—a delicious twist on the classic fried rice, where quinoa replaces rice, and cauliflower adds a hearty, nutritious base. Packed with a colorful array of vegetables and protein, this grain-free dish promises a flavorful and satisfying meal that's both wholesome and delicious.

Ingredients:

For the Cauliflower Rice:

• One medium-sized cauliflower, grated or processed into rice-sized pieces

• One tablespoon of sesame oil

• Two cloves garlic, minced

• One tablespoon ginger, grated

• 2 cups mixed vegetables (carrots, peas, corn, bell peppers), diced

• 1 cup cooked quinoa

• Two eggs, lightly beaten

- Three green onions, chopped
- Two tablespoons of low-sodium soy sauce
- One tablespoon of rice vinegar
- Salt and pepper to taste

Instructions:

1. Preparing Cauliflower Rice:

- Grate or process the cauliflower into rice-sized pieces using a food processor.

2. Sautéing Cauliflower Rice:

- In a large skillet or wok, heat sesame oil over medium heat.

- Add minced garlic and grated ginger, sautéing for about 1 minute until fragrant.

3. Cooking Vegetables:

- Add the mixed vegetables to the skillet and stir-fry until they are crisp-tender.

4. Incorporating Cauliflower and Quinoa:

- Add the cauliflower rice and cooked quinoa to the skillet, stirring well to combine.

5. Making a Well for Eggs:

- Push the cauliflower and quinoa mixture to the sides of the skillet, creating a well in the center.

6. Cooking Eggs:

- Pour the beaten eggs into the well and scramble them until cooked through.

7. Combining Ingredients:

- Mix the scrambled eggs with the cauliflower and quinoa

mixture.

8. Adding Green Onions:

• Stir in chopped green onions.

9. Seasoning:

• Drizzle the soy sauce and rice vinegar over the mixture. Stir well to distribute the flavors evenly.

10. Adjusting Seasoning:

• Season with salt and pepper to taste.

11. Serving:

• Serve the Cauliflower Fried Rice with Quinoa hot.

12. Enjoying:

• Delight in this grain-free version of fried rice, relishing the combination of cauliflower, quinoa, and vibrant vegetables.

Note:

• Customize the dish with your favorite protein, such as diced chicken, shrimp, or tofu.

• For added freshness, garnish with additional chopped green onions or a sprinkle of cilantro.

Nutrition Information (per serving):

• Calories: 250

• Protein: 10g

• Carbohydrates: 40g

• Fat: 8g

• Fiber: 8g

• Sugar: 6g

- Sodium: 500mg

SPELT FLOUR BANANA BREAD

Banana Bread Description: Indulge in the wholesome goodness of our Spelt Flour Banana Bread—a delightful twist on the classic treat. Made with nutty spelled flour, ripe bananas, and a touch of warmth from cinnamon, this banana bread brings comfort to your taste buds and adds a nutritious element to your baking repertoire.

Ingredients:

• 2 to 3 ripe bananas, mashed (about 1 cup)

• 1/3 cup melted coconut oil or vegetable oil

• 1/2 cup maple syrup or honey

• One large egg

• One teaspoon of vanilla extract

• 1 1/2 cups spelt flour

• One teaspoon baking soda

• 1/4 teaspoon salt

• 1/2 teaspoon ground cinnamon (optional)

• 1/2 cup chopped nuts (walnuts or pecans), optional

• Additional banana slices for topping (optional)

Instructions:

1. Preparing the Oven:

• Preheat your oven to 350°F (175°C). Grease a 9x5-inch loaf pan.

2. Mashing Bananas:

• Mash the ripe bananas with a fork or potato masher in a large mixing bowl until smooth.

3. Adding Wet Ingredients:

• Add melted coconut oil or vegetable oil, maple syrup or honey, egg, and vanilla extract to the mashed bananas. Mix until well combined.

4. Sifting Dry Ingredients:

• Sift together spelled flour, baking soda, salt, and ground cinnamon in a separate bowl.

5. Combining Wet and Dry:

• Add the dry ingredients to the wet ingredients and stir until just combined. Avoid overmixing.

6. Adding Nuts (Optional):

• Fold in the chopped nuts if using.

7. Pouring into Pan:

• Pour the batter into the greased loaf pan, spreading it evenly.

8. Topping with Banana Slices (Optional):

• Optionally, place banana slices on top of the batter for a decorative touch.

9. Baking:

• Bake in the preheated oven for 55-65 minutes or until a toothpick inserted into the center comes out clean or with a few moist crumbs.

10. Cooling:

• Allow the banana bread to cool in the pan for about 10 minutes before transferring it to a wire rack to cool completely.

11. Slicing and Enjoying:

• Once cooled, slice the Spelt Flour Banana Bread and enjoy the nutty and flavorful goodness.

Note:

• Ensure that your bananas are ripe for the best sweetness and flavor.

• Customize the bread by adding chocolate chips or dried fruit for extra texture and sweetness.

Nutrition Information (per slice):

• Calories: 180

• Protein: 3g

• Carbohydrates: 24g

• Fat: 8g

• Fiber: 3g

• Sugar: 11g

• Sodium: 150mg

CHAPTER SIX

Lean Protein Recipes

Grilled Chicken and Vegetable Skewers

Skewer Description: Elevate your summer grilling experience with these Grilled Chicken and Vegetable Skewers, a colorful and flavorful feast featuring marinated grilled chicken, vibrant bell peppers, and red onions. Perfect for a barbecue or a simple outdoor gathering, these skewers promise a delicious combination of smoky, charred goodness and juicy, tender bites.

Ingredients:

For the Marinade:

• 1/4 cup olive oil

• Two tablespoons of soy sauce

• One tablespoon honey

• Two cloves garlic, minced

• One teaspoon paprika

• One teaspoon dried oregano

• Salt and black pepper to taste

For the Skewers:

• 1.5 lbs boneless, skinless chicken breasts, cut into 1-inch cubes

• Two bell peppers (assorted colors), cut into chunks

• One large red onion, cut into chunks

• Wooden or metal skewers (if using wooden skewers, soak them in water for at least 30 minutes)

Instructions:

1. Preparing Marinade:

• Whisk together olive oil, soy sauce, honey, minced garlic, paprika, dried oregano, salt, and black pepper to create the Marinade.

2. Marinating Chicken:

• Place the chicken cubes in a resealable plastic bag or a shallow dish. Pour half of the Marinade over the chicken, ensuring each piece is coated. Reserve the remaining Marinade for basting.

3. Marinating Time:

• Marinate the chicken in the refrigerator for at least 30 minutes to allow the flavors to infuse.

4. Preparing Skewers:

• Preheat the grill to medium-high heat.

• Thread the marinated chicken cubes, bell pepper chunks, and red onion chunks onto the skewers, alternating between ingredients.

5. Basting:

• Brush the skewers with the reserved Marinade for extra flavor while grilling.

6. Grilling:

• Grill the skewers for 10-15 minutes, turning occasionally, until the chicken is fully cooked and has a nice char.

7. Checking Doneness:

• Ensure the chicken reaches an internal temperature of 165°F (74°C).

8. Resting:

• Allow the skewers to rest for a few minutes before

serving.

9. Serving:

• Serve the Grilled Chicken and Vegetable Skewers hot, garnished with fresh herbs if desired.

10. Enjoying:

• Dive into these succulent skewers, savoring the harmony of marinated grilled chicken and the vibrant sweetness of bell peppers and red onions.

Note:

• Experiment with additional vegetables like cherry tomatoes or mushrooms for extra variety.

• These skewers are great on their own or paired with a side of rice or a fresh salad.

Nutrition Information (per serving - 2 skewers):

• Calories: 300

• Protein: 30g

• Carbohydrates: 15g

• Fat: 14g

• Fiber: 3g

• Sugar: 9g

• Sodium: 600mg

TURKEY AND QUINOA MEATBALLS

Meatball Description: Enjoy a nutritious twist on traditional meatballs with our Turkey and Quinoa Meatballs. Crafted with lean ground turkey, quinoa, and a blend of herbs and spices, these meatballs offer a burst of flavor without sacrificing health. Whether baked or grilled, they are a versatile addition to your meals—perfect for pairing with pasta, salads, or as a tasty appetizer.

Ingredients:

- 1 lb lean ground turkey

- 1 cup cooked quinoa, cooled

- 1/4 cup grated Parmesan cheese

- 1/4 cup breadcrumbs (whole wheat or gluten-free)

- 1/4 cup fresh parsley, finely chopped

- Two cloves garlic, minced

- One teaspoon dried oregano

- One teaspoon of dried basil

- 1/2 teaspoon onion powder

- 1/2 teaspoon paprika

- Salt and pepper to taste

- One large egg, beaten

- Cooking spray (if baking)

Instructions:

1. Preparing Quinoa:

- Cook quinoa according to package instructions. Allow it to cool.

2. Preheating Oven or Grill:

- Preheat your oven to 400°F (200°C) if baking, or preheat your grill.

3. Mixing Ingredients:

- Combine ground turkey, cooked quinoa, Parmesan cheese, breadcrumbs, chopped parsley, minced garlic, dried oregano, dried basil, onion powder, paprika, salt, and pepper in a large mixing bowl.

4. Binding with Egg:

- Add the beaten egg to the mixture, ensuring it binds everything together.

5. Forming Meatballs:

- With clean hands, gently mix the ingredients until well combined.

- Shape the mixture into meatballs, approximately 1 to 1.5 inches in diameter.

6. Baking Method:

- If baking, place the meatballs on a baking sheet lined with parchment paper.

- Bake in the preheated oven for 15-20 minutes or until the

internal temperature reaches 165°F (74°C).

7. Grilling Method:

• If grilling, place the meatballs on preheated grill grates.

• Grill for about 10-15 minutes, turning occasionally, until fully cooked.

8. Checking Doneness:

• Ensure the internal temperature of the meatballs reaches 165°F (74°C).

9. Resting:

• Allow the meatballs to rest for a few minutes before serving.

10. Serving:

• Serve the Turkey and Quinoa Meatballs hot, either on their own or with your favorite sauce.

11. Enjoying:

• Relish these lean and flavorful meatballs, appreciating the wholesome combination of turkey and quinoa.

Note:

• Customize the herbs and spices to suit your taste preferences.

• These meatballs are excellent for meal prep and can be stored in the refrigerator for several days.

Nutrition Information (per serving - 4 meatballs):

• Calories: 250

• Protein: 28g

• Carbohydrates: 15g

• Fat: 9g

- Fiber: 2g
- Sugar: 1g
- Sodium: 350mg

LENTIL AND TURKEY CHILI

Chili Description: Warm up your evenings with a bowl of our hearty Lentil and Turkey Chili—a flavorful blend of lean ground turkey, nutritious lentils, tomatoes, and a medley of spices. Packed with protein, fiber, and rich flavors, this chili is a comforting and satisfying dish that's perfect for chilly nights or as a crowd-pleasing meal during gatherings.

Ingredients:

- 1 lb lean ground turkey

- 1 cup dry brown lentils, rinsed and drained

- One large onion, diced

- Three cloves garlic, minced

- One bell pepper (any color), diced

- One can (14 oz) diced tomatoes, undrained

- One can (14 oz) crushed tomatoes

- One can (14 oz) black beans, drained and rinsed

- One can (14 oz) kidney beans, drained and rinsed

- Two tablespoons of tomato paste

- One tablespoon of chili powder

• One teaspoon of ground cumin

• One teaspoon of smoked paprika

• 1/2 teaspoon dried oregano

• 1/2 teaspoon ground coriander

• Salt and black pepper to taste

• 2 cups low-sodium chicken or vegetable broth

• Olive oil for sautéing

Instructions:

1. Sautéing Aromatics:

• Heat a bit of olive oil over medium heat in a large pot. Sauté the diced onion, minced garlic, and diced bell pepper until softened.

2. Browning Turkey:

• Add the lean ground turkey to the pot and cook until browned, breaking it apart with a spoon as it cooks.

3. Incorporating Spices:

• Stir in the chili powder, ground cumin, smoked paprika, dried oregano, ground coriander, salt, and black pepper. Cook for 1-2 minutes until the spices are fragrant.

4. Adding Lentils and Tomatoes:

• Add the rinsed lentils, diced tomatoes, crushed tomatoes, black beans, kidney beans, and tomato paste to the pot. Stir well to combine.

5. Pouring Broth:

• Pour in the chicken or vegetable broth. Bring the chili to a boil, then reduce the heat to low, cover, and simmer for about 30-40 minutes or until the lentils are tender.

6. Checking Seasoning:

• Taste and adjust the seasoning if needed. Add more salt, pepper, or spices according to your preference.

7. Serving:

• Serve the Lentil and Turkey Chili hot, optionally topped with shredded cheese, chopped green onions, or a dollop of Greek yogurt.

8. Enjoying:

• Enjoy this hearty and wholesome bowl of chili, savoring the combination of lean turkey, lentils, and spices.

Note:

• Customize the spice level by adjusting the chili powder and black pepper amount.

• This chili can be made ahead of time and freezes well for convenient future meals.

Nutrition Information (per serving):

• Calories: 350

• Protein: 28g

• Carbohydrates: 40g

• Fat: 9g

• Fiber: 15g

• Sugar: 6g

• Sodium: 600mg

BAKED LEMON HERB COD

Cod Description: Elevate your seafood experience with our Baked Lemon Herb Cod—a light and flavorful dish that features tender cod fillets baked to perfection with a zesty lemon and herb marinade. This recipe offers a burst of freshness and a symphony of herbs that perfectly complement the delicate flavor of cod. Enjoy a healthy and delicious meal that's quick to prepare and delightful to savor.

Ingredients:

• Four cod fillets (6 ounces each), fresh or thawed if frozen

• Zest and juice of 1 lemon

• Two tablespoons fresh parsley, chopped

• One tablespoon of fresh dill, chopped

• Two cloves garlic, minced

• Two tablespoons of olive oil

• Salt and black pepper to taste

• Lemon slices for garnish

• Optional: 1 teaspoon of Dijon mustard for added tanginess

Instructions:

1. Preparing the Marinade:

• In a small bowl, combine the lemon zest, lemon juice, chopped parsley, chopped dill, minced garlic, olive oil, salt, and black pepper.

• If using Dijon mustard, whisk it into the Marinade for added flavor.

2. Marinating the Cod:

• Place the cod fillets in a shallow dish or a resealable plastic bag.

• Pour the lemon herb Marinade over the cod, ensuring each fillet is well-coated. Marinate for at least 20-30 minutes to let the flavors infuse.

3. Preheating the Oven:

• Preheat the oven to 400°F (200°C).

4. Baking the Cod:

• Place the marinated cod fillets on a baking sheet lined with parchment paper.

• Bake in the preheated oven for 12-15 minutes or until the cod is opaque and flakes easily with a fork.

5. Checking Doneness:

• Ensure the internal temperature of the cod reaches 145°F (63°C).

6. Resting:

• Allow the cod to rest for a few minutes before serving.

7. Garnishing:

• Garnish the Baked Lemon Herb Cod with additional chopped herbs and lemon slices.

8. Serving:

• Serve the cod fillets hot, accompanied by your favorite side dishes or a fresh salad.

9. Enjoying:

• Delight in the light and zesty flavors of the Baked Lemon Herb Cod, appreciating the perfect balance of citrus and herbs.

Note:

• This recipe works well with other white fish varieties like haddock or tilapia.

• For a complete meal, consider serving the cod over a bed of quinoa or with steamed vegetables.

Nutrition Information (per serving):

• Calories: 200

• Protein: 25g

• Carbohydrates: 2g

• Fat: 10g

• Fiber: 1g

• Sugar: 0g

• Sodium: 300mg

TOFU AND BROCCOLI STIR-FRY

Stir-Fry Description: Elevate plant-based culinary adventures with our Tofu and Broccoli Stir-Fry. In this vibrant and flavorful dish, tofu and Broccoli take center stage in a delectable ginger-soy sauce. Quick, nutritious, and bursting with Asian-inspired flavors, this stir-fry is a delightful way to enjoy a satisfying and veggie-packed meal.

Ingredients:

For the Stir-Fry:

• One block (14 ounces) of firm tofu, pressed and cubed

• 3 cups broccoli florets

• Two tablespoons vegetable oil (for Cooking)

• Two green onions, sliced (for garnish)

• Sesame seeds (for garnish, optional)

For the Ginger-Soy Sauce:

• Three tablespoons soy sauce (reduced sodium)

• Two tablespoons water

• One tablespoon of rice vinegar

• One tablespoon of maple syrup or agave nectar

• One tablespoon of fresh ginger, minced

• Two cloves garlic, minced

• One teaspoon of cornstarch (optional for thickening)

Instructions:

1. Pressing Tofu:

• Press the tofu to remove excess moisture. Place the tofu between two kitchen towels and press under a heavy object (such as a plate with cans on top) for 20-30 minutes.

2. Preparing Sauce:

• Whisk together soy sauce, water, rice vinegar, maple syrup or agave nectar, minced ginger, and minced garlic in a small bowl. If you prefer a thicker sauce, whisk in cornstarch.

3. Cubing Tofu:

• Once pressed, cut the tofu into bite-sized cubes.

4. Stir-Frying Tofu:

• Heat vegetable oil in a wok or large skillet over medium-high heat.

• Add the cubed tofu and stir-fry until golden brown on all sides.

5. Adding Broccoli:

• Add broccoli florets to the wok and continue to stir-fry for 3-4 minutes until the Broccoli is crisp-tender.

6. Incorporating Sauce:

• Pour the ginger-soy sauce over the tofu and Broccoli. Stir to coat evenly.

7. Simmering:

• Allow the stir-fry to simmer for an additional 2-3 minutes, allowing the flavors to meld.

8. Checking Seasoning:

• Taste and adjust the seasoning if needed. Add more soy sauce or sweetener, according to your preference.

9. Serving:

• Serve the Tofu and Broccoli Stir-Fry over rice or noodles.

10. Garnishing:

• Garnish with sliced green onions and sesame seeds if desired.

11. Enjoying:

• Dive into this flavorful and nutritious stir-fry, relishing the harmony of tofu, Broccoli, and the zesty ginger-soy sauce.

Note:

• Customize the stir-fry with additional veggies like bell peppers, snap peas, or carrots.

• For added protein, sprinkle with crushed peanuts or cashews before serving.

Nutrition Information (per serving):

• Calories: 250

• Protein: 15g

• Carbohydrates: 20g

• Fat: 13g

• Fiber: 6g

• Sugar: 6g

• Sodium: 600mg

EGG WHITE OMELETTE WITH SPINACH AND FETA

Omelette Description: Start your day on a nutritious note with our Egg White Omelette with Spinach and Feta— a light and fluffy omelet that combines the freshness of sautéed Spinach with the savory richness of feta cheese. Packed with protein and low in calories, this breakfast option is delicious and a wholesome way to kickstart your morning.

Ingredients:

• Four large egg whites

• 1 cup fresh Spinach, chopped

• Two tablespoons of feta cheese crumbled

• One tablespoon of olive oil

• Salt and black pepper to taste

• Optional: Chopped fresh herbs (such as parsley or chives) for garnish

Instructions:

1. Preparing Spinach:

• In a small pan, heat olive oil over medium heat. Add

chopped Spinach and sauté until wilted. Set aside.

2. Whisking Egg Whites:

• In a bowl, whisk the egg whites until they form soft peaks. Season with salt and black pepper to taste.

3. Cooking Egg Whites:

• Heat a non-stick skillet over medium heat. Pour the whisked egg whites into the skillet, spreading them evenly.

4. Adding Spinach and Feta:

• Spoon the sautéed Spinach onto one-half of the cooking egg whites.

• Sprinkle crumbled feta cheese over the Spinach.

5. Folding Omelette:

• Once the edges of the egg whites start to set, carefully fold the other half of the omelet over the spinach and feta filling.

6. Finishing Cooking:

• Continue cooking for 1-2 minutes or until the egg whites are fully set.

7. Checking Doneness:

• Ensure the omelet is cooked through, with no runny egg whites.

8. Garnishing:

• Slide the omelet onto a plate. Garnish with chopped fresh herbs if desired.

9. Serving:

• Serve the Egg White Omelette hot, either on its own or with whole-grain toast or a side of fresh fruit.

10. Enjoying:

• Delight in this light and flavorful breakfast, savoring the combination of fluffy egg whites, sautéed Spinach, and the creamy richness of feta.

Note:

• Customize the omelet by adding diced tomatoes, mushrooms, or bell peppers for extra freshness and variety.

• If you prefer a richer flavor, consider mixing whole eggs and egg whites.

Nutrition Information (per serving):

• Calories: 150

• Protein: 20g

• Carbohydrates: 3g

• Fat: 7g

• Fiber: 1g

• Sugar: 1g

• Sodium: 400mg

CHICKEN AND VEGETABLE QUINOA BOWL

Quinoa Bowl Description: Savor the goodness of our Chicken and Vegetable Quinoa Bowl. This wholesome and satisfying dish combines grilled chicken's protein, quinoa's nourishment, and the richness of roasted vegetables. Tying it all together is a delightful drizzle of tahini, adding a creamy and nutty finish to this nutritious bowl.

Ingredients:

For the Quinoa Bowl:

• 1 cup quinoa, rinsed

• 2 cups water or vegetable broth (for cooking quinoa)

• 1 lb boneless, skinless chicken breasts, grilled and sliced

• 2 cups mixed vegetables (e.g., bell peppers, zucchini, cherry tomatoes), roasted

• One tablespoon of olive oil

• Salt and black pepper to taste

For the Tahini Drizzle:

• 1/4 cup tahini

• Two tablespoons of lemon juice

- One clove garlic, minced

- Two tablespoons water (to thin the sauce)

- Salt to taste

Instructions:

1. Cooking Quinoa:

- In a medium saucepan, combine quinoa and water or vegetable broth. Bring to a boil, then reduce heat, cover, and simmer for 15-20 minutes or until quinoa is cooked and water is absorbed. Fluff with a fork.

2. Grilling Chicken:

- Season the chicken breasts with salt and black pepper.

- Grill the chicken until fully cooked, about 6-8 minutes per side, depending on thickness.

- Allow the chicken to rest for a few minutes before slicing.

3. Roasting Vegetables:

- Preheat the oven to 400°F (200°C).

- Toss the mixed vegetables with olive oil, salt, and black pepper.

- Spread the vegetables on a baking sheet and roast for 20-25 minutes or until they are tender and slightly caramelized.

4. Preparing Tahini Drizzle:

- Whisk together tahini, lemon juice, minced garlic, and water in a small bowl until smooth. Add salt to taste.

5. Assembling Quinoa Bowl:

- Layer cooked quinoa, grilled chicken slices, and roasted vegetables in serving bowls.

6. Drizzling Tahini:

• Drizzle the tahini sauce over the quinoa bowl.

7. Garnishing (Optional):

• Garnish with fresh herbs, such as chopped parsley or cilantro, for added freshness.

8. Serving:

• Serve the Chicken and Vegetable Quinoa Bowl warm.

9. Enjoying:

• Enjoy this nutritious and balanced bowl, savoring the combination of quinoa, grilled chicken, roasted vegetables, and the creamy tahini drizzle.

Note:

• Customize the bowl with your favorite vegetables, or add avocado slices for extra creaminess.

• This recipe is versatile; you can substitute the chicken with grilled tofu or chickpeas for a vegetarian version.

Nutrition Information (per serving):

• Calories: 450

• Protein: 30g

• Carbohydrates: 45g

• Fat: 18g

• Fiber: 8g

• Sugar: 4g

• Sodium: 400mg

SHRIMP AND AVOCADO SALAD

Salad Description: Elevate your salad experience with our Shrimp and Avocado Salad—a refreshing medley of succulent shrimp, creamy avocado, and crisp mixed greens, all harmonized by a zesty citrus dressing. Packed with vibrant flavors and nutrients, this Salad is perfect for a light and satisfying meal that's as delicious as it is nourishing.

Ingredients:

For the Salad:

- 1 lb large shrimp, peeled and deveined

- Two avocados, sliced

- 6 cups mixed salad greens (e.g., Spinach, arugula, romaine)

- 1 cup cherry tomatoes, halved

- 1/4 cup red onion, thinly sliced

- 1/4 cup fresh cilantro, chopped (optional)

- Salt and black pepper to taste

For the Citrus Dressing:

- 1/4 cup olive oil

- Two tablespoons of fresh lime juice

- One tablespoon of fresh orange juice

- One teaspoon of honey or agave nectar

- One teaspoon of Dijon mustard

- One clove garlic, minced

- Salt and black pepper to taste

Instructions:

1. Cooking Shrimp:

- Season the shrimp with salt and black pepper.

- In a pan, heat a bit of olive oil over medium-high heat.

- Cook the shrimp for 2-3 minutes per side or until they turn pink and opaque. Set aside.

2. Assembling Salad:

- Combine the mixed greens, sliced avocados, halved cherry tomatoes, thinly sliced red onion, and cooked shrimp in a large salad bowl.

3. Preparing Citrus Dressing:

- Whisk together olive oil, fresh lime juice, fresh orange juice, honey or agave nectar, Dijon mustard, minced garlic, salt, and black pepper in a small bowl.

4. Drizzling Dressing:

- Drizzle the citrus dressing over the Salad.

5. Tossing Salad:

- Gently toss the Salad to coat the ingredients with the dressing.

6. Garnishing (Optional):

- Garnish the Salad with fresh cilantro for an added burst of flavor.

7. Serving:

• Divide the Shrimp and Avocado Salad among serving plates.

8. Enjoying:

• Enjoy this refreshing and nourishing Salad, savoring the combination of succulent shrimp, creamy avocado, and the citrusy zing of the dressing.

Note:

• Customize the Salad by adding your favorite nuts or seeds for crunch.

• This Salad is perfect for meal prep; store the dressing separately until ready to serve.

Nutrition Information (per serving):

• Calories: 400

• Protein: 25g

• Carbohydrates: 20g

• Fat: 28g

• Fiber: 10g

• Sugar: 7g

• Sodium: 400mg

CHAPTER SEVEN

Hydration Recipes

Cucumber and Mint Infused Water

Infused Water Description: Stay cool and hydrated with our Cucumber and Mint Infused Water—a revitalizing blend that transforms simple Water into a refreshing and flavorful beverage. With the natural crispness of cucumber and the refreshing aroma of fresh mint leaves, this infused Water is a delightful way to stay hydrated throughout the day without added sugars or artificial flavors.

Ingredients:

• One cucumber, thinly sliced

• One handful of fresh mint leaves

• 8 cups water (filtered or still)

• Ice cubes (optional)

Instructions:

1. Preparing Ingredients:

• Wash the cucumber thoroughly. Slice it thinly, keeping the skin on for added flavor.

• Rinse the fresh mint leaves under cold Water.

2. Assembling Infused Water:

• In a large pitcher, combine the cucumber slices and fresh mint leaves.

3. Adding Water:

• Pour 8 cups of Water over the cucumber and mint in the pitcher.

4. Infusing:

• Allow the Water to infuse for at least 2-4 hours. For a more robust flavor, you can refrigerate it overnight.

5. Serving:

• Strain the infused Water to remove cucumber slices and mint leaves, or leave them in for a more intense flavor.

6. Adding Ice (Optional):

• If desired, add ice cubes to the infused water before serving.

7. Pouring and Enjoying:

• Pour the Cucumber and Mint Infused Water into glasses and enjoy the refreshing and subtle flavor.

Note:

• Feel free to experiment with other additions like lemon slices, berries, or a splash of sparkling water for variation.

• This infused Water is an excellent alternative to sugary drinks, providing a burst of natural flavors.

Benefits:

• Cucumber adds hydration and a mild, crisp flavor.

• Mint provides a refreshing aroma and may aid digestion.

Tip:

• Reuse the cucumber and mint for a second batch of infused Water. The flavors may be less intense, but it's a sustainable way to enjoy the infusion.

Hydration Benefits:

• Infused Water can encourage increased water intake, promoting overall hydration.

• The refreshing taste can make drinking water more enjoyable, particularly for those who find plain Water less appealing.

COCONUT WATER SMOOTHIE

Smoothie Description: Transport yourself to a tropical paradise with our Coconut Water Smoothie—a hydrating blend that combines the natural sweetness of pineapple and mango with the refreshing taste of coconut water. Add a handful of spinach for a nutritious twist, creating a smoothie that satisfies your taste buds and provides a healthy dose of vitamins and minerals.

Ingredients:

• 1 cup coconut water

• 1 cup pineapple chunks (fresh or frozen)

• 1/2 cup mango chunks (fresh or frozen)

• One handful of fresh spinach leaves

• Ice cubes (optional)

• Optional: Chia seeds or flaxseeds for added nutrition

Instructions:

1. Gathering Ingredients:

• Peel and chop the pineapple and mango into chunks if using fresh fruit.

2. Assembling in Blender:

• Combine the coconut water, pineapple chunks, mango

chunks, and a handful of fresh spinach leaves in a blender.

3. Blending:

• Blend the ingredients until smooth and creamy. If a thicker consistency is desired, add ice cubes and blend again.

4. Checking Consistency:

• Check the consistency and adjust by adding more coconut water if needed.

5. Optional Additions:

• Consider incorporating a tablespoon of chia seeds or flaxseeds into the blend for added nutrition. Blend again to combine.

6. Pouring and Serving:

• Pour the Coconut Water Smoothie into a glass.

7. Garnishing (Optional):

• Garnish with a slice of pineapple or a sprinkle of chia seeds for a decorative touch.

8. Enjoying:

• Sip and savor this tropical delight, appreciating the hydrating and nutritious coconut water, pineapple, mango, and spinach blend.

Note:

• Adjust the sweetness by adding more or less mango and pineapple according to your taste preferences.

• Feel free to customize the smoothie with additional fruits like banana or kiwi for variety.

Benefits:

• Coconut Water: Hydrating and rich in electrolytes.

• Pineapple: Packed with vitamins and enzymes, known for its sweet and tangy flavor.

• Mango: A good source of vitamin C and adds natural sweetness.

• Spinach: Provides a boost of vitamins and minerals without altering the flavor significantly.

Nutrition Information (approximate):

• Calories: 150

• Carbohydrates: 36g

• Fiber: 5g

• Sugars: 28g

• Protein: 3g

• Fat: 1g

• Sodium: 200mg

TURMERIC AND GINGER HERBAL TEA

Herbal Tea Description: Experience the comforting embrace of our Turmeric and Ginger Herbal Tea—a warm infusion that brings together the earthy notes of turmeric, the zesty kick of ginger, and a touch of sweetness from Honey. This soothing Tea not only delights your senses but also offers potential health benefits from the anti-inflammatory properties of turmeric and the digestive aid of ginger.

Ingredients:

• One teaspoon of ground turmeric or 1-inch fresh turmeric, sliced

• One teaspoon of fresh ginger, grated or 1-2 slices

• One tablespoon honey (adjust to taste)

• One tea bag or one teaspoon of leaf tea (black or green Tea works well)

• 2 cups hot Water

Instructions:

1. Preparing Ingredients:

• If using fresh turmeric, peel and slice it into thin rounds. Grate the fresh ginger or cut it into thin pieces.

2. Boiling Water:

• Bring 2 cups of Water to a boil.

3. Infusing Turmeric and Ginger:

• Add ground turmeric or fresh turmeric slices and grated ginger in a teapot or heatproof pitcher.

4. Pouring Hot Water:

• Pour the hot water over the turmeric and ginger.

5. Steeping:

• Place the tea bag or loose-leaf Tea into the hot Water. Allow the Tea to steep for 5-7 minutes or longer for a more robust flavor.

6. Straining (Optional):

• If using loose-leaf Tea, strain the Tea to remove the leaves. If using a tea bag, remove the bag.

7. Adding Honey:

• Stir in Honey to sweeten the Tea. Adjust the amount based on your preference.

8. Serving:

• Pour the Turmeric and Ginger Herbal Tea into cups.

9. Enjoying:

• Sip and savor the warmth of this herbal Tea, letting the soothing blend of turmeric and ginger comfort your senses.

Note:

• Experiment with the quantities of turmeric, ginger, and Honey to find the balance that suits your taste.

• Feel free to add a splash of lemon juice for a citrusy twist.

Benefits:

• Turmeric: Known for its anti-inflammatory properties.

• Ginger: Aids digestion and adds a zesty flavor.

• Honey: Provides natural sweetness and may have soothing properties.

Potential Health Benefits:

• This herbal Tea may help with inflammation and digestion, making it a soothing choice for various occasions.

BERRY AND BASIL INFUSED ICED TEA

Iced Tea Description: Quench your thirst with our Berry and Basil Infused Iced Tea—an excellent and flavorful blend that marries the sweetness of mixed berries with the aromatic essence of fresh basil leaves. This refreshing iced Tea is a delightful way to stay cool on warm days while enjoying the vibrant and natural infusion of berries and herbs.

Ingredients:

• Two black tea bags or two tablespoons of leaf black tea

• 1 cup mixed berries (strawberries, blueberries, raspberries)

• 1/4 cup fresh basil leaves

• Two tablespoons honey or agave nectar (adjust to taste)

• Ice cubes

• Lemon slices for garnish (optional)

Instructions:

1. Brewing Black Tea:

• Brew black Tea by steeping the tea bags or loose-leaf tea in hot water for 3-5 minutes. Remove the tea bags or strain the loose-leaf Tea.

2. Muddling Berries and Basil:

• Muddle the mixed berries and fresh basil leaves in a pitcher to release their flavors.

3. Adding Honey:

• Add honey or agave nectar to the muddled berries and basil. Adjust the sweetness to your liking.

4. Pouring Tea:

• Pour the freshly brewed black Tea over the muddled mixture.

5. Stirring:

• Give the mixture a gentle stir to combine the Tea with the berries, basil, and sweetener.

6. Refrigerating:

• Place the pitcher in the refrigerator to chill for at least 2 hours or until thoroughly chilled.

7. Straining (Optional):

• Strain the iced Tea to remove the berry and basil remnants if you prefer a smoother texture. Alternatively, leave them for added visual appeal and flavor.

8. Adding Ice:

• Before serving, add ice cubes to the pitcher for a frosty finish.

9. Garnishing (Optional):

• Garnish individual glasses with lemon slices for an extra burst of freshness.

10. Serving:

• Pour the Berry and Basil Infused Iced Tea into glasses.

11. Enjoying:

• Sip and relish the refreshing blend of berries, basil, and black Tea in this cooling and delightful iced beverage.

Note:

• Experiment with different berry combinations based on your preferences.

• Add a few whole berries and basil leaves to each glass to enhance the visual appeal before serving.

Benefits:

• Berries: Packed with antioxidants and natural sweetness.

• Basil: Adds a unique and aromatic flavor, plus potential health benefits.

• Black Tea: Contains antioxidants and provides a base for the infusion.

LEMON WATER WITH CHIA SEEDS

Lemon Water Description: Elevate your hydration routine with our Lemon Water with Chia Seeds. This refreshing and nutritious drink combines Lemon's zesty kick with chia seeds' added benefits. This simple yet rejuvenating elixir keeps you hydrated and provides a burst of energy and essential nutrients.

Ingredients:

• One lemon, sliced

• Two tablespoons chia seeds

• 4 cups water (filtered or still)

• Ice cubes (optional)

• 1-2 tablespoons honey or agave nectar (optional for sweetness)

Instructions:

1. Slicing Lemon:

• Wash the Lemon thoroughly and slice it into thin rounds.

2. Preparing Chia Seeds:

• In a small bowl, combine chia seeds with 1/2 cup of Water. Stir well and let them sit for 10-15 minutes until they form a gel-like consistency.

3. Assembling Lemon Water:

• In a pitcher, combine the lemon slices with 4 cups of Water.

4. Adding Chia Seeds:

• Pour the soaked chia seeds into the lemon water. Stir gently to distribute the seeds.

5. Sweetening (Optional):

• If desired, add honey or agave nectar to sweeten the lemon water. Adjust the sweetness to your liking.

6. Adding Ice (Optional):

• Drop ice cubes into the pitcher for a chilled and refreshing beverage.

7. Stirring:

• Give the lemon water a final stir to ensure that the chia seeds are evenly distributed.

8. Serving:

• Pour the Lemon Water with Chia Seeds into glasses.

9. Enjoying:

• Sip and enjoy this hydrating elixir, relishing the combination of citrusy Lemon and the unique texture of chia seeds.

Note:

• Chia seeds add a fun texture to the drink but can be omitted if you prefer a smoother beverage.

• Customize the sweetness level according to your taste preferences.

• This drink can be enjoyed immediately or refrigerated for

a more chilled experience.

Benefits:

• Lemon: Rich in vitamin C and adds a refreshing citrus flavor.

• Chia Seeds: Provide omega-3 fatty acids, fiber, and a unique gel-like texture.

• Honey or Agave Nectar: Adds natural sweetness.

Nutrition Information (approximate):

• Calories: 40

• Carbohydrates: 8g

• Fiber: 6g

• Sugars: 1g

• Fat: 2g

• Protein: 1g

• Sodium: 5mg

WATERMELON AND MINT SLUSHIE

Slushie Description: Beat the heat with our Watermelon and Mint Slushie. This refreshing and hydrating concoction combines the natural sweetness of frozen watermelon with the refreshing kick of fresh mint. This vibrant slushie is not only a delightful way to cool down on a hot day but also a tasty way to enjoy the flavors of summer.

Ingredients:

• 4 cups frozen watermelon cubes

• 1/4 cup fresh mint leaves

• One tablespoon of honey or agave nectar (optional for added sweetness)

• 1 cup cold Water

• Ice cubes (optional for a thicker slushie)

Instructions:

1. Freezing Watermelon:

• Cut fresh watermelon into cubes and freeze them for at least 4 hours or until solid.

2. Assembling in Blender:

• InCombinehe frozen watermelon cubes, fresh mint leaves,

and cold Water.

In a blender3. Blending:

• Blend the ingredients until smooth and slushie-like. If the mixture is too thick, you can add more cold Water.

4. Sweetening (Optional):

• Taste the slushie and add honey or agave nectar if you desire additional sweetness. Blend again to incorporate.

5. Checking Consistency:

• If you prefer a thicker slushie, you can add ice cubes and blend until desired consistency is reached.

6. Pouring:

• Pour the Watermelon and Mint Slushie into glasses.

7. Garnishing (Optional):

• Garnish with a sprig of fresh mint or a watermelon wedge for a decorative touch.

8. Enjoying:

• Sip and enjoy the calm and refreshing taste of this Watermelon and Mint Slushie, perfect for beating the summer heat.

Note:

• Experiment with the mint quantity to achieve your preferred level of minty freshness.

• Customize the sweetness level according to your taste preferences.

Benefits:

• Watermelon: High water content and natural sweetness.

• Mint: Adds a cooling sensation and a burst of flavor.

• Honey or Agave Nectar: Optional for those who prefer a sweeter slushie.

Nutrition Information (approximate):

• Calories: 80

• Carbohydrates: 20g

• Fiber: 2g

• Sugars: 16g

• Fat: 0g

• Protein: 1g

• Sodium: 5mg

CONCLUSION

I n conclusion, the journey through Polymyalgia Rheumatica (PMR) reveals a complex interplay of symptoms, medical interventions, and lifestyle adjustments. This chronic inflammatory condition presents unique challenges, impacting the lives of individuals and often requiring a multifaceted approach to management.

As we've explored, the management of PMR extends beyond traditional medical treatments, with emerging attention given to the potential impact of diet on symptoms and overall well-being. While there is no one-size-fits-all "PMR diet," the significance of making informed dietary choices to support overall health and manage inflammation cannot be understated.

Understanding the inflammatory nature of PMR prompts a closer look at anti-inflammatory foods and nutrients that may offer relief. Incorporating a diet rich in fruits, vegetables, whole grains, and lean proteins while limiting processed foods and potential triggers is a step towards fostering an environment that supports the body in its battle against inflammation.

Nevertheless, the key to successfully navigating the complexities of PMR lies in collaboration between individuals and their healthcare providers. Personalized treatment plans, including dietary considerations, should be crafted with the guidance of medical professionals who understand the intricacies of this condition.